Turn Off Your Age

About the author

Elsye Birkinshaw is the director and founder of the Seminars of Self-Awareness Center, conducting highly successful classes throughout the United States, including regular programs for California State University Extension, now being expanded worldwide. These classes have proved to be effective in behavior modification in relation to problems of compulsive eating, smoking, inferiority feelings, emotional problems, and the problems of aging.

Seminars of Self-Awareness has now initiated a new phase called The Image Consultants, which includes telephone consultations and correspondence studies in various areas of living, such as: Learning to Be the Image of Success, Time Management, and Dressing for Success.

Turn Off Your Age

A Guide to Youthful Long Life

By Elsye Birkinshaw

Author of Think Slim–Be Slim
Director, Seminars of Self Awareness Center
Lecturer, California State University Extension

Published by

Woodbridge Press Publishing Company
Santa Barbara, California 93111

No medical or health advice is given in this book as a prescription for any specific person or case, because individual conditions and requirements differ. Where personal health is concerned, and particularly in the presence of a medical history or of symptoms of any kind, competent medical advice should be obtained.

Published and Distributed by
Woodbridge Press Publishing Company
Post Office Box 6189
Santa Barbara, California 93111

Published simultaneously in the United States and Canada
Printed in the United States of America

Library of Congress Cataloging in Publication Data

Birkinshaw, Elsye.
  Turn off your age.

  1. Aged—Care and hygiene. 2. Longevity.
3. Aging. I. Title.
RA777.6.B57   613'.0438   79-27693
ISBN 0-912800-75-5

Table of Contents

CHAPTER 1

Turn Off Your Age

Deep within all of us, in the very center of our being, is a longing. In the beginning it is wordless, but as time goes on, it begins to form itself into feelings, then a definite desire. Finally the cry wells up inside of us, growing in intensity as the years race by: *"Why must I get old?"*

At one time or another, most of us have had the wish to look and act youthful indefinitely. As the years slip by, most of us eventually dismiss this idea as mere wishful thinking and accept the alternative, "Everyone grows old, so I might just as well grow old gracefully."

No diseases of the aged

But this is not true! No one has to either look or act old unless they deliberately choose to do so. Even medical science has come to this conclusion in recent years after extensive research. The American Medical Association has published a booklet called "A New Concept of Aging," which states that there are

7

no "diseases of the aging." To rephrase this statement, there do not seem to be any diseases that result specifically because of the mere passing of a certain number of years. "We have no right to assume," the report continues, "that the shaky hand, the wobbly step and the narrowing of horizons are inevitable at a certain age. They are caused by a lack of physical and mental exercise, *not* by the passage of a certain number of years." American Medical Association: Committee on Aging, Council and Medical Service of A.M.A. (Proceedings of House of Delegates, January, 1968 [emphasis supplied].)

We have been tricked into believing a great many things from the moment we were born. As newborn infants, our minds are as clean and blank as a slate, but the moment we arrive into this world, the mesmerism and hypnotism begin. Perhaps we were told that sitting in a draft would cause a cold, but now science has proved this is not so. We may have been fooled into believing that if we are around infectious diseases we will also be infected, but this is not always the case. Doctors and nurses are continually surrounded by diseases in hospitals and there is no evidence that they have more infectious diseases than anyone else. The belief that we must get old just because the years roll by is just another one of the many erroneous theories we have been taught to accept.

Concepts forced upon us

Our world is composed of these mental concepts the cultural process has led us to believe. Most of the concepts and beliefs we live by were instilled in us as children—erroneous statements such as "Put on your boots or you'll catch cold." We knew we would not catch a cold, but what choice did we have but to obey? Now research has proved that putting on boots does not necessarily keep one from having colds. There were hundreds of other erroneous statements, many of which put fear in our hearts. "Eat everything on your plate or you'll never grow as big as Daddy." That was not a true statement, was it? All of these statements were made to discipline, to make us conform to our society. Unfortunately, they also had the sad side benefit of installing mountains of fear within our minds.

As children we rebelled silently against such stupid things as putting on our boots when it was cold. Others rebelled a bit more openly and protested in loud cries, but to no avail. As children surrounded by giant adults, we had to do as we were told. So throughout our childhood we were coerced, threatened, disciplined, and given rewards when we finally did conform.

Then something strange happened—the rebellion of our teen-age years. Our parents no longer knew how to cope with their children. The threats, the punishments, the disciplines no longer seemed to work. It suddenly appeared as if these teenagers had completely overthrown all of the earlier training that parents had so carefully given them. It appeared that the fear-whip that had been so useful as a control no longer had any effect. The teenagers rebelled openly against old and worn-out concepts such as putting on their boots so they wouldn't get sick or eating everything on their plates so they'd get as big as Daddy. They already towered five inches over Daddy. They were finally realizing that many things they had been taught were not true.

But sadly, when the teen years were over, those old and worn-out concepts were finally accepted because there was nothing to put in their place. When the formerly rebellious teenagers had children of their own, they also were taught, "Put on your boots or you will catch cold." "Eat everything on your plate so you'll grow big as Daddy."

Thus a vast structure of erroneous concepts has come to be regarded as firm truths within us and we live by them. Right or wrong, we live by these beliefs because we *know* beyond a shadow of a doubt they are true. We have nothing to put in their place.

Belief is the key

There is however, a secret that very few people are aware of. It is not the erroneous concept that we live by. No, it is the *belief* in the concept that we live by. That is where the power of the concept is, the *belief* in it. *What you believe to be true is the law you live by!* If you believe that wearing boots will keep you from catching cold, then you will never catch cold as long as you are wearing them. If you go out without wearing them, you probably will catch a cold. But the boots themselves do not have a secret potion that is resistant to cold germs. No, it is only the belief in the magic of the boots that prevents miserable colds, *not the boots themselves.*

So it is with the beliefs, attitudes, and concepts you

were taught during childhood. They are true to you if you believe they are true, not necessarily because of the concepts themselves.

A student during one of my seminars on the East Coast had a very difficult time. As a child she had been taught that females are not as intelligent as males and thus should be subservient to men. An idealized male image was presented to her throughout her entire childhood, which she believed. When she finally married, her husband of course could not be like the ideal picture she had been fooled into believing. She went through a terrible inner conflict because the picture of "truth" she had been taught cracked right through the middle. She was finally able to realize that both men and women have faults and are not perfect, but they all try to do the best they can. It was fortunate this happened to this student at an early age because through this realization she was also able to see that the "aging myth" she had been taught was not true. Now, at age 52, she lives an energetic life, very successful in her field, with an appearance of being in her late 30s.

Your life is a mirror

Your mental concepts and beliefs, whether true or not, make your world and operate in your life as truths, making your life whatever it is, good or bad. Be aware that your life is a mirror of your inner beliefs.

Look around. Are you happy with your life and environment? If so, then your beliefs must be positive and operating in a positive way for you. If you have an unhappy, depressing life, this is not your fate, but is because you have accepted certain erroneous beliefs as truth and they are now operating in your life. You can change the beliefs, and in so doing you will automatically change your world.

The concept of aging, which is so coyly explained as "something that happens to everyone after the passing of a certain number of years," is also an erroneous belief and concept that has been accepted by the majority of the world as a truth.

If we accept this as a mental concept and truth, we will make it happen. "Dad died of a heart attack at 45, so I guess it will happen to me." "Premature grey hair runs in our family so I'm sure I'll have grey hair soon." "Mother started getting wrinkles at age 50, so I'll also have them then." "I'll probably get old and senile around 75 because Daddy was pretty active until then but that was it." And so on.

Interestingly enough, there are also other people who say things like, "I come from a long-lived family, so guess I'll be around for a long time too." "My folks all lived to be in their late 90s and some even over 100, very energetic and active. I'm sure I will have the same experience." "Grandma finished first in a marathon jogging race when she was 79; sure glad our family has that kind of vitality."

People who have been exceptions

There are people here and there throughout the world who have been trailblazers, proving to us it is not absolutely necessary to grow old and feeble!

In China, the famous herbalist, Li Chung Yun,

lived to be 256 years of age, dying in 1933. The *New York Times* reported this remarkable man, whose age was apparently confirmed by the Chinese government after a thorough investigation had been made by the head of Chang-Tu University. Li outlived 23 wives and was living with the 24th at the time of his death. He was a vegetarian who attributed his longevity to herbs, ginseng and Fo-ti-Tieng (an herb found in the jungle of the eastern tropics). Li was said to have had a calm and serene attitude toward life.

There have been other outstanding exceptions to this old-age myth—men and women who are miracles of mental, physical, artistic, and creative energy far beyond the "three score and ten."

Titian, the great artist born in 1477 in Italy, produced some of his greatest paintings in his 90s. Roscoe Pound, a well-known legal educator, wrote five volumes on American jurisprudence after he was 86. Thomas Parr, a farmer who lived in England, not only threshed grain at 130 years of age and lived to be 153, but he was accused and tried for committing a sexual offense at the age of 102. Drankenberg, a native of Denmark, lived to be 146 years of age, and at 130 fell in love and wanted to marry a 16-year-old girl. (She turned him down.) The Italian baron Baravicino de Capellis married at age 84 for the fourth time and had seven children before he died at about 107. Peter Albrecht, an Englishman, had seven children after he remarried at 85 and then lived to be 123.

In our own time there have been many talented and "ageless" people—such as Pablo Picasso, Pablo Casals, Bernard Baruch, Winston Churchill, Charlie Chaplin, Golda Meir, and Grandma Moses—great artists, musicians, and statesmen. All of these people did some of their greatest work in their later years. There was also Larry Lewis, who at age 105 felt he was too young for retirement. He had tried retiring as a waiter at the St. Francis Hotel in San Francisco, but after a few weeks of boredom went back to work. Marie Cardoza took up horseback riding at age 75, but later rode a bicycle because she said she could never find any riding horses with spirit. At least with a bicycle she could go as fast as she wanted to. In Pacific Grove, California, I met a member of the Polar Bear Club who was over 85 years of age. One of the club requirements is to take a dip in the ocean every day, summer or winter. The ocean around Pacific Grove is chilly in the summer and in the winter it is truly cold.

There are others who have lived long and productive lives, full of energy, such as Gloria Swanson, Will and Ariel Durant, Marlene Dietrich, Arthur Fiedler, Artur Rubenstein, and many others too numerous to list. We all know of such people who have seen the passing of a great many years, but who still live a full and active life with their appearance belying their years.

What is the secret?

The important thing to remember when you read about these amazing people is not to simply say to yourself, "Isn't that wonderful. I certainly hope at that age I can do as well." No, the important thing is that you ask yourself, "What secret have these people found? What principle of life are they using that has allowed them to *turn off their age?*" These people and many more like them have proved that there is no law of life that tells you that at a certain age you *must* grow old.

Corporations, industries, doctors, and even the government try to set a certain age as "retirement age." This implies that 65 or 70 is the sad number that tells you that you are out of the race of life, that you'd better take it easy, go fishing, slow down, get out of the rat race. Don't believe them! No, the people that show youthfulness way beyond the so-called retirement years have all proved there is no hard and fast law of life that you must wear out and deteriorate just because of the passing of a certain number of years.

A lie has been forced upon you, the belief that you *must* grow old, decrepit, and feeble. The world has been saying for generations, "Everyone grows old," and you have been led to believe this lie. Do not believe "them." "They" do not know what they are talking about. Awaken out of your "sleep" and realize that you do not have to grow old and feeble, that this is only a myth. There have been many people throughout the ages who have proved that the aging process is not necessary. We have their histories and documentary evidence of how they thought and what they did, so we can follow their example.

The first question is, "Why do we grow old when it is not necessary? Why do we allow the erroneous belief of aging to deceive us until we follow the aging pattern of all the generations?"

New babies are born with a clean "mental slate" on which can be imprinted either positive or negative beliefs and concepts. Most babies are born expecting love, beauty, and perfection, but after a short time the negative world beliefs are imprinted over the perfection of the infant's being, thus distorting the image of perfection.

Your body reflects your beliefs

The mental image you have of yourself is the blueprint of your body, so very quickly your body will show the distorted image you have in your mind. The body actually changes and becomes imprinted with the world beliefs of old age. There are also other factors that bring about body changes. Pollution, radiation, illness, and tensions all distort the original perfection. These factors actually interfere with the body cells' ability to reproduce themselves as perfect replicas. Thus these cell mutations are misshaped, causing symptoms of wrinkled skin, sagging muscles, liver spots, etc.—the signs of "old age."

This is where the process of aging begins, first the imprinting of your mind with erroneous beliefs, then the distortion of your body cells right to the very nucleus of the cell. Eventually your body shows wrinkles, discolorations, sagging muscles, and all the other symptoms of old age. This is the process of aging.

Can this aging process be slowed?

Can it be halted?

Can it be reversed?

Yes—on all questions!

There are indeed ways this can be accomplished, so now let us begin to *"turn off your age!"*

CHAPTER 2

Dissolve Your Erroneous Mental Concepts

The first step in turning off your age is recognition: recognition of the fact that you have been given false information. This false information began in your infancy when all the relatives and friends began to ask, "How old is the baby?" The word *old* begins even then to have a special significance. It means the developing and maturing of various physical functions. The baby begins first to recognize its parents, then learns to smile, eat, walk, and so on. These are all positive things because the parents usually are very proud of their offspring's progress. If the baby is especially fast in learning to walk, mother will say proudly, "Johnny was walking by the time he was nine months old." Quickly Johnny gets the idea that it is good to learn things in a hurry because he gets

17

praise and positive "vibrations" from everyone around him. So time begins to accelerate for him. Each time he learns something ahead of other children in his age group, he receives praise. This works very well in childhood. To most children time passes very slowly. They cannot wait until they are 12, or 16, or 21 years old.

Then something very strange begins to happen when Johnny is in his early 20s. The word *old* begins to have another meaning for him. He looks around him and realizes that the older one gets, the more physical functions seem to deteriorate. His grandfather, who was so active at age 50, now just sits around at age 65 after retirement. His father, who used to smash a tennis ball four days a week, now has changed to a less active form of recreation. So naturally, the assumption is that if Johnny's father and grandfather slowed down at those ages, he will also.

You may think that the error in thinking of the word *old* began at that moment, but, no, it had already started from the moment Johnny was born. The false concept of "time" had already begun. The concept of time that most of us entertain means a steady progression toward the inevitable end of old age. But this is not necessarily true.

Time is relative

Albert Einstein proved that time is only relative. Many of us have had experiences that have also proved that time is only relative. When you have had a very enjoyable experience with people you like, then the time span of an hour seemed like a few moments. On the other hand, when we are doing something we do not enjoy, the time span of an hour may seem like a year. So the concept we call "time" is only in relation to whatever we happen to be doing and feeling at any given moment.

When Johnny was very young, the word *old* meant good, because he received praise for all of his accomplishments. When he began to mature, the word *old* had frightening implications because he began to relate to his father and grandfather and their activities, thinking he would also be doing the same thing at that same age.

This is the first erroneous mental concept that must be corrected. "Time," or the passing of a certain number of years, does *not* have to mean the inevitable steady progress toward a period called "old age" with all of its implications of slowing down physically and mentally and enjoying life less.

At this point you must *consciously* begin to recognize that you have false information; you may even call it "garbage" in your mind. You must do more than just read this and think, "Hey, this is great." No, the word *consciously* means much more than that. It means you must actually work out a plan of action so this new information will penetrate the subconscious layers of your mind and make the false concepts begin to peel off. This process can be likened to the peeling away of one layer of an onion skin, as the Hindus so aptly used this illustration. One layer is hardly noticeable, but by the time you have peeled away ten or twenty layers, you can see a definite difference.

So how do you do this, consciously?

We are very fortunate to have by now the results of

a great deal of research with the mind and how it functions, so we can formulate a plan of action. Very little was known about the inner world of the mind as recently as fifteen years ago. There is still a great deal more to be discovered, but with the knowledge we have, it has been possible to formulate a definite plan of action that will turn off your age.

Persistence is the secret

There is only one secret to this process, and it is not that you must be a genius, or be wealthy, or even have a great talent. No, the only secret involved is *persistence*. This alone will accomplish anything you want to do.

Through the research done with the human mind, we have learned that the mind works in a certain way. Because of this, there is a formula that has been found to work in exactly the same way each time it is used. It has been used successfully not only in turning off your age, but in many other areas of life.

The first step to be taken in a sequence of mental steps is the reconditioning of your subconscious mind and erasing the false information that you have been storing deep in the lower "layers." Recognize it for what it is. Think back to your earlier years. How many times when you had a birthday did friends ask you, "How old are you today?" Then, perhaps kiddingly, they would follow this with a remark such as "You're really getting up there now." Unfortunately, even if someone treats it as a joke, your mind takes this literally and accepts these false statements. Then because your mind controls your body, the belief that you are getting older begins to start the process of deterioration and the body shortly begins to show the effects. When you look in the mirror and see a wrinkle or two, this immediately reinforces the statement and you believe that you are truly getting old. Then, because you believe this so firmly, soon it begins to show more and more and then you are on a merry-go-round of aging that seems impossible to get off.

A simple technique

There is a way to keep your mind from accepting these statements even though you cannot keep people from saying them. A very simple technique is to say to yourself the words, "*cancel, cancel.*" This will immediately erase the effects of any negative statements so they will not lodge in your subconscious mind.

But how do you get rid of the negative statements that have already been accepted into your mind throughout all the years? We know that your subconscious mind functions in somewhat the same way that a computer functions. This does not mean that you are a machine. What it does mean is that you have a marvelous "machine" that can be used, a fabulous instrument greater than any instrument man has yet invented.

In fact, it is this instrument that is responsible for all of the great inventions. There have been so-called geniuses throughout the ages that have known how to use the mind correctly and have come forth with great ideas. These ideas have always been there, but

it took a person who knew how to use the mind correctly to tap these energies and come forth with them.
For example, electricity has been around for millions
of years, but it took Thomas Edison, who knew how to
use his mind correctly, to show us how to use it. How
did he use his mind? Not by will power, forcing his
mind to pump out ideas. No, he took many catnaps
and always had a listening attitude, and his ideas
came from within—within himself, from the depths
of his inner self.

Our mind is the last frontier

This is the last frontier we have yet to explore, and
each person must do it for himself. This exploration
will never be a group project because there is no way
one person can reach inside another to bring forth the
great creativity of that person's mind. Other people
can show you the way. People who have already trod
that path can show you how to avoid the pitfalls and
point out the guideposts, but no one but you can
actually do the work. It *must* be done in order to shed
these false beliefs of old age, sickness, negativity, and
depression.

These are all erroneous concepts that have been
forced upon us by common beliefs. All through the
ages we see examples of false beliefs that people accepted until an enterprising individual proved them
to be false. For hundreds of years people believed the
earth was flat until Columbus and others proved this
to be wrong. Many more years went by before the
Wright brothers proved that birds were not the only
creatures that could soar in the sky.

From the beginning of time, false beliefs and erroneous concepts have ruled the lives of millions of people until they were proved to be wrong. These beliefs have been interwoven with other concepts until the whole network of lies and deceits were so believable that people had no choice except to believe and thus construct their lives upon these mires of quicksand.

Now the time has come to break through one more of these false beliefs—the belief in old age, so that the truth can now begin to operate instead of the false concept that enslaves us.

What you must do now is to learn exactly how your mind works. Then you will begin to see how these pieces of false information have shaped your ideas and attitudes and thus formed your habits. Your life is composed of 95 percent firmly entrenched habits, over which you have little or no control until you recognize them and set out deliberately to change them.

Recognition and action

The two prime factors are *recognition and action*. With these two factors you can shape your life and future into anything you wish. The rules to be followed in order to erase the "garbage" in your mind are surprisingly simple. *Persistence* is the only real secret to this process because there will be times when you get discouraged, when your progress will not be as rapid as you would like it to be. Understanding how the mind functions is one of the keys to overcoming the inertia that may set in at times.

One student reached a time of discouragement and was able to recognize that his inertia was simply another of the tricks that the mind plays on us from time to time. He redoubled his efforts and in a very short time overcame the inertia and went on to outstanding success. If you find that nothing is happening for awhile, always review your procedures. My students have always discovered that if they are not achieving their goals, it is not the procedure itself that is at fault, but that many times a small but important step has been left out.

You are setting into motion a law of the mind that works exactly as any other physical law works. For example, when you plant a seed you must give it proper light, water, and nourishment, and then it grows. If you neglect to give it water, it does not help to get discouraged; the only thing that will help is water. So it is with the law of your mind: it always works if properly executed. When you know how it works, you can set it into operation exactly as if you were planting a seed. You would plant it in good soil, give it the correct amount of moisture and light, and would exercise a certain amount of patience or faith and wait until you begin to see the result of your actions—a tiny bit of green sprout. *Remember, you are the law in operation itself.*

Plant your goal in your mind

The law of nature and the law of the mind work in exactly the same way. By setting the goal, which is like the seed, into the pliable substance of your mind, you can then nourish it with the actions that are described and explained in later chapters of this book. Then exercise patience and faith exactly as if you had planted a seed until you begin to see the first tiny bit of change.

When the goal or change that you have decided on is something like turning off your age, all three aspects of a person—physical, mental-emotional, and spiritual—must be changed.

You are a total person, not purely physical or purely mental or purely spiritual, but a combination of all three, making a total fulfilled whole. So you will be working on all three levels. However, the deliberate actions need to be taken on only the physical and mental-emotional levels. The spiritual results will follow. But always keep in mind that you are a great deal more than a physical body or emotions or a mind. Your true being is of such magnitude that at the present you cannot conceive of it. As you work along these lines you will begin to get a glimpse into your true nature.

Now let us see how the inner workings of your subconscious mind operate.

CHAPTER 3

The Inner Workings of Your Mind

How does your mind work? This question has long engaged the interest of enterprising people. However, the method by which your mind works is a very recent discovery. It was only with the invention of the now commonplace computer that this question was illuminated.

What a paradox it is that man should invent the computer and then discover that his own mind is "programmed" in much the same way as the machine he invented. Of course, the human mind is vastly more complex than any computer that has yet been built. It also has an extra ingredient that no computer will ever have, and that is awareness of itself. You are aware that you are you, and no machine can ever be aware of itself. In essence, you have a billion-dollar computer waiting for you to use, sitting on your

27

shoulders, with all of the inner workings of the most advanced machine ever built. But there is more: in addition, you also have creativity, imagination, and a potential for greatness that no computer has ever had.

Habits are programmed

But remember that your habits, which compose 95 percent of your life, are programmed much like any computer program. Your habits are completely automatic. You do not even think about the habitual things you do. Your habits are centered in the subconscious level of your mind. Think of your habits for a moment. Perhaps you bite your fingernails, for example. Do you ever consciously make a decision to bite your nails? Of course not; you probably do not even notice that you are doing it.

Can you see that your habits control you? Can you see how your negative habits can hold you in bondage, make you a prisoner of your own mind?

You have only to choose the *correct* goals, take the *correct* action and you can have anything, be anything and do anything you wish. It's as simple as that. I won't promise it will always be easy to do, but it is a very simple process. First your conscious mind sets a goal, you take the appropriate actions, and in as short a time as twenty-one days, you have formed a new habit. With this book, choose the goal of youthful maturity and that is what we will work toward.

Principles to follow

There are certain specific principles that must be used, and they must be used in an exact order. The principles, which are listed below, will be discussed in much greater detail in subsequent chapters.

The first principle is *desire*. You must want to do something in order for anything to happen. The greater the intensity of desire, the more quickly your goal will be achieved. For example, the story is told of the great philosopher who was approached by a prospective student. The student said he wanted knowledge above all things. The philosopher said he understood, and took the student out into the river and held his head under the water. The student, of course, struggled to get a breath after a few minutes. After what seemed like an eternity to him, he was at last allowed to lift his head out of the water and take a breath. Puzzled by this treatment, he asked the great man why he'd treated him in this manner. The philosopher asked the student what he wanted more than anything else while he was under the water. The student replied that he'd naturally wanted a breath of air above all else. The wise man nodded his head, and said, "When you desire knowledge as much as you wanted that breath of air, then you will receive it." The greater your desire for anything, the faster you will achieve your goal. You probably already have this desire or you would not be reading this book.

The second principle is to *set a goal*. There are certain specific ways to set goals, which must be followed in exact order. These are discussed in detail in a later chapter.

The third principle is to use the great *creative process* of your mind, "the fantasizing process," or mental imagery, and to use it correctly.

The fourth principle is to use the *mirror image technique* so you can feel *worthy* of remaining youthful indefinitely. Many people do not feel as if they are worthy of achieving great and marvelous things. These people are their own worst enemies.

One of the students in the "Turn Off Your Age" seminar found this to be true when she had problems in following certain steps in the procedure. Whenever she tried to write down her goals and to use the mirror technique, something always seemed to interfere, such as having to do things for her children and her husband before she could sit down and do something for herself. It happened so regularly and so often that she was finally forced to do some deep inner searching. She then realized that her self-concept was so low that in order to accept herself at all, she had to put aside her own feelings and wishes completely. This caused great frustration because she could not do the things she wanted to do until all her other duties were finished. By that time she was either too tired, or it was late into the night.

Through the seminar she finally realized that she had been conditioned as a child to believe that a wife and mother must first care for her family before she can do anything for herself. This is a wonderful attitude if it makes you sincerely self-fulfilled and happy. However, this student also wanted a little time for herself, and this caused the feelings of frustration. She had to first raise her self-concept so she could take an hour or two each day for her desires without feeling so guilty that her subconscious mind could not allow her to do so.

Your mind has a way of playing tricks on you. Many times it is hard to sort out your true wishes. These are the "sly little foxes" of your mind.

There was a very interesting example of this in a recent weight-loss seminar. A student was very much overweight and thought he wanted to lose the excess weight. Consciously, this student thought this way. But when we went into a relaxation exercise, his true subconscious feelings were brought to the surface.

One of the statements students make to themselves during this exercise is, "I now enjoy low-calorie nutritious foods and am satisfied with only one-half of what I usually eat." At that moment the student suddenly had a very violent coughing and sneezing fit and was brought out of relaxation immediately. This same reaction happened five times, so finally he was able to see that in reality he did not want to give up his rich foods. He wanted to keep right on eating.

You must be very alert as to the real reasons buried deep in your subconscious mind when you seemingly are always thwarted from achieving your desires and goals. Ask yourself at this point, "What is keeping me from reaching my goal?" Do some soul searching; remember back to your early childhood. The reason is *always* within yourself, even though many times it appears that there are outside influences, such as the two examples given above. Your own mind can be your own worst enemy unless you dissolve these negative erroneous conditionings, which nine times out of ten began in early childhood.

The fifth and one of the most important principles

is *deep relaxation*. This is very important because there is no other way to reach the deeper levels of your subconscious mind except through deep inner relaxation. You must reach your subconscious mind, not only to bring to the surface many of the "sly little foxes," but also to erase negative programming and imprint positive conditioning. You were conditioned in this manner as a child, so we must use exactly the same method to bring about positive changes.

These are the five simple techniques that can and will bring about a tremendous change in your life. Each one will be discussed in great detail in the following chapters because there are specific reasons for each one and exact ways to use them.

Work with the total person

You are a total person, so you must work with the total person. You must work with your physical body, your mind-emotions, and your spirituality. It never works if you only keep your physical body in good shape through diet and exercise; or if you only use your mind to picture yourself being youthful; or even if you only realize the spiritual principle to "know" that you were meant to have eternal youth.

This is a physical and mental world conditioned by spiritual principles, so it is necessary to combine all three of these aspects of living, and to combine them in the correct sequence. This can be compared to a three-legged stool: if one leg is broken, the stool will not stand up. If all of the aspects of living are not used in their natural sequence, you will topple into old age.

The correct way for your mind to function is for

your conscious mind to have the desire and set the goal and for your subconscious mind to achieve the goal through various methods. Your subconscious mind has control of all your involuntary bodily functions such as your digestive system, breathing, heart, etc. So the correct order is for the conscious mind to make the decision or goal and for the subconscious mind to get the involuntary body functions working to bring it about. This method can be likened to your conscious mind as being the executive and giving the orders, and your subconscious mind being the employee and carrying out the orders.

However, because of your early negative childhood training, it now works in reverse. Your conscious mind has the desire, but your subconscious mind actually sets the goal based on the "garbage" in your subconscious. Before you realize what is happening, you are doing something in exact opposition to your desire. This happens many times in trying to break the smoking habit or trying to lose weight. The desire is strong to achieve these positive habits, but the "garbage programming" in the subconscious mind prevents many people from reaching their conscious goals. The only way to deal with this is to erase the "garbage."

You have set habit patterns in your subconscious mind, etched in your brain cells, that work automatically in firmly entrenched habits. You must consciously be aware of what is happening and also *consciously* begin to change these patterns, or engrams, before you can see any results. The engrams in your brain cells regarding the so-called aging process are very deeply grooved, so deep that they are almost the fiber of your being.

Time has no power

The very first thing you must realize is that there is no power in the concept of time or years except the power you yourself give to it. If you look at a calendar and bemoan that you're a year older, you're giving power to a concept. The calendar certainly does not know how many years you've been around. Only you give importance to that. Never think of yourself as getting older, think of yourself as getting "newer."

Just as there is no power in food except the power you give it, there is no power in concepts unless you give power to them. What you believe in is the only power that operates in your life. For example, many people believe that if they eat a piece of cake with 500 calories they will gain several pounds, but there are just as many people who firmly believe that no matter what they eat they will never gain an ounce. So the power is not in the piece of cake, but what each person believes that piece of cake will do to him. Because the belief is in the mind, that is where the power is.

Your mind controls your body

Your mind controls your body. Your body does not have the ability to do anything without instructions from your mind. Try this simple test to demonstrate this to yourself. Sit in a chair, look at your feet, and ask yourself, "Do my feet have the ability to walk across the room by themselves, or do my hands have any power in themselves to pick up a toothpick?" Of course not. Nothing will happen unless you give instructions through your mind.

If your mind tells your body what to do, what is in

your mind? Your mind is composed of habitual responses, attitudes, and beliefs that you were taught in early childhood. You were conditioned or programmed with these habits, attitudes, and beliefs as a very young child, and you were unable to keep yourself from learning a great deal of wrong information, bad habits, and negative beliefs.

One of the most firmly entrenched beliefs is that of growing old as the years roll by and you have birthday after birthday. On each birthday you were asked, "How old are you today?" After being asked this question many times, it finally becomes an automatic habit to think that with each year and each birthday you are getting older and older.

Body cells renew

Your body is not getting older each year, because each of your body cells (with a few exceptions) is constantly being renewed. There is not a cell in your renewing cells that has been in your body over seven years, no matter what your age is. Many research scientists believe that the body is a completely self-renewing instrument that should continue renewing much longer than it does. So it appears that our problem is not in our body cells being renewed, but in giving instructions to our mind to allow our body to self-renew.

In other words, with our wrong beliefs and wrong thinking, we have jammed up the self-renewing machinery of our minds. On the mental level, we must become aware of this so it can be stopped. On the physical level, there are certain foods that will allow the body cells to reproduce in a perfect pattern, thus overcoming the effects of the constant pollution of our environment.

Dr. Benjamin S. Frank of New York City has done research over a period of twenty years to prove that not only can the aging process be slowed, but it can be halted and even reversed. He says that one of the most obvious effects of aging is the wrinkling of the skin.

"In aging skin there is a decrease in elasticity and a thinning due to loss of fat and water. Lines and wrinkles in the face and hands become more prominent. The backs of the hands are highly visible indicators of age. They become shiny, and spotted with brownish, pigmented areas. Why do these changes occur? Because the cells which contain the blueprints for the formation of the various organs are tired and worn and no longer able to maintain the pattern they inherited."

The process appears to be due to the acceptance by the subconscious mind that at 50, 60, or 70 one must grow old, plus the environmental pollution we are bombarded with twenty-four hours a day. This sounds very depressing, but by using a combination of the mental exercises, physical actions, and diets, and remembering at all times that we are also spiritual beings, the aging process can be overcome to an impressive degree. You will be able to slow the aging process, halt it, and actually reverse it.

Many students in our seminars have proved that there is no necessity for allowing themselves to grow old. One of our students proved this not only to herself but also to her husband. She came into the class looking fifteen years older than her forty years. Her children no longer needed her as they once had, and she found herself without a goal. She had an increasing feeling of uselessness and was allowing herself to grow old. As she progressed throughout the seminar, she realized that she was the one who had been giving power to the old age process. After the seminar was over, she called long distance a few months later and said her husband had remarked that he had never seen such a change in anyone. He was also interested in using the procedure outlined in this book and was already making remarkable progress.

Let us break the chains of wrong beliefs and attitudes that up to this moment have allowed you to age.

CHAPTER 4

Break The Chains That Bind You To The Age Myth

The age myth is the chain that binds you to the negative, so-called truths you have accepted into your subconscious mind. Your entire life is regulated and restricted by this limitation. Do some serious soul-searching, and you will undoubtedly find that very little of what you accept as "right" is also accepted as "right" throughout the world. For example, the society you now live in does not approve of running around half-nude, and yet in some tropical societies this is not only accepted, but necessary because of climatic conditions.

"Truths" may be illusions

Many of the so-called truths that our lives are built upon are like the shifting sands of the desert that change when the winds blow. So this reveals the interesting premise that many of the truths you live by, and have built your life on, are illusions. In other words, many so-called truths are really just beliefs, convictions, rules of the society you live in, restrictions of a religious faith, and early childhood conditioning. In other words, the prison you have made for yourself consists merely of suggestions impressed upon you and everyone else by the world and the society we live in. They can be changed the moment you consciously perceive this fact. Recognize that the limitations you have placed on yourself are not only untrue, but can be changed now, at this very moment!

One spiritual principle many people believe is that mankind has been created in the image of God and He has never created anything that is not perfect. If you believe this premise, how can you account for the fact that you are growing old or getting sick, depressed, worried, or fearful? Can you believe that God—spiritual principle, universal life, call it any name you please—made a mistake? Of course not! Most of us will agree on this point. So we must confront our own errors, mistaken ideas and worn-out concepts that seem to cause most of the problems in our life.

The problem is within ourselves

If we can agree with the reasoning that the problem lies within us, it becomes simply a matter of changing ourselves within. If it depended upon our outside environment, we would be lost because we cannot change much of that. But we can change ourselves. Change yourself within and you change your own world. It's that simple!

The first step in dissolving the myth of old age is to recognize that it is not true! You do not have to grow old unless you set about deliberately to do so.

The next step is to consciously and deliberately begin to erase the wrong ideas you have about the so-called aging process. You will have to do this the first thing upon arising every day because you will be bombarded all during the day with the false concepts that will once again pull you into the quicksand of belief in old age if you are not *consciously aware* of this process. This is the secret, to be consciously aware. It is not enough to say once or twice as you are reading this book, "I like this idea and I want to believe it." No, you must work with it every day, all during the day, always knowing consciously that you are doing so.

A mental exercise

The first thing upon awakening in the morning, before you even get out of bed, you must discipline your mind by refusing to accept the world beliefs of aging. As you are awakening, begin to say to yourself:

"Nothing can enter my mind from the outside because my mind is an instrument through which I function. It is not an instrument through which somebody else functions, or through which wrong world beliefs function. My mind is an instrument given to me just as my body is given to me. As I keep my body inviolate, so I keep my mind inviolate, free from the erroneous world beliefs of age. I do not permit my mind to be used by suggestion, by outside influence, or by outside opinions or theories. I make my mind an instrument for the truth and only the truth. I recognize that age is only a world belief and I do not choose to accept the world belief of "age." I choose to be ageless!

Do this every morning before you get out of bed and the very last thing at night just as you are drifting off to sleep. You may find after you have been practicing this mental exercise for a few days that you are even saying this to yourself while sleeping. Several students have mentioned that they have awakened during the night saying this to themselves. If this happens, it means that your subconscious mind has begun to operate in a positive way with these words and it will be but a short period before the mistaken beliefs about aging are all but erased.

You can also be influenced by ideas and subconscious thoughts from your outside environment of which you may not even be aware. An illustration of how you may be involuntarily influenced is an experiment that was conducted some years ago. On a motion picture screen was flashed a message directing the audience to buy popcorn. The words were flashed too quickly for the conscious minds of the people in the theater to perceive them, but they were impressed upon the subconscious mind. During intermission sales of popcorn significantly increased—even though the audience had no awareness of having been exposed to a "selling" message. This is called "subliminal perception," and it operates without anyone having a conscious awareness of it. Unfortunately, a great many advertisements in the mass media operate in almost the same way. This is one of the reasons you have many wrong ideas or "garbage" in your mind. The acceptance of these beliefs make you a victim of them.

Freeze your age

The simple mental exercise you can do each morning and evening that was described above will protect you from the effects of subliminal perception in any form. The second very important thing to be accomplished through the practice of this mental exercise is that it will *freeze your age* at the point it is now. It will not advance beyond this point the moment you begin the conscious realizing and saying these words to yourself each morning and evening. The secret is that you must be aware of what you are doing. By being aware, you are disciplining your mind instead of your mind disciplining you.

One student said she always woke up with a negative or depressed feeling in the morning until she had practiced this mental exercise for several weeks. Then she began to experience feelings of joy and well-being upon awakening. At first when she opened her eyes she would feel that it was just another dreary day, but as she began to say the exercise and it slowly seeped through the deeper layers of her mind, she could just feel the negative feeling begin to lift. When she was finished, she'd get out of bed with a joyous feeling. (At first she said it many times before even getting out of bed.) You may not experience a happy feeling at first. It takes at least twenty-one days to form the simplest of habits. That is what you are doing by practicing this exercise: you are changing a negative habit to a positive one. So be patient and just keep on doing it until you experience a change of feeling.

The next important step after the freezing of your age is to halt it. This is done by the realization of the total person you are: that you know you are a physical, mental-emotional, spiritual person. Chapters 5, 6, 7, and 8 will deal with the physical level. It is always the easiest level to begin with because the results of the physical actions can be seen at once. The mental exercises are more abstract and a knowledge of how the mind works is necessary before a student will realize how important they are.

The spiritual level will take care of itself because it is always present, but has been hidden from view because of the negative mental-emotional conditions of the mind. It can be likened to a window that has been left unwashed for many years. It is impossible to see inside until the window glass has been washed. The moment you begin to change the negative mental conditions and feelings to more positive ones, your spiritual level will come into view. Do not concern yourself with that at the present.

Let us start, then, at the physical level and begin the transition from belief in the law of age to a realization that it is not a hard and fast law, but only a belief, and beliefs can always be changed.

CHAPTER 5

Attaining the Prize: Youthful Maturity

What happens to your body as the years roll by and you begin to show facial wrinkles, tissue sagging, liver spots, etc? When you see these outward visible signs of age, recognize that they are often the result of negative subconscious thinking. What the mind thinks shows up in the body sooner or later.

Look in the mirror

Look at yourself in the mirror very closely. What you see in the mirror is the direct outward result of the habitual thinking you have been doing throughout your lifetime. If you have been in the habit of worrying, holding resentful thoughts, harboring grudges, having negative thoughts of any kind the *major* part of your day, then sooner or later it will show outwardly on your face and body. Notice that it is the *majority* of the time. A worry or negative thought now and then is of no concern. After all, no one is perfect.

It is important for you to do some deep soul-searching and to be very honest with yourself. Ask yourself, "Do I habitually hold negative thoughts for much of my day?"

You may notice examples of negative thinking all around you. Look at your friends, relatives, and neighbors. Which ones are always voicing fears, worrying, being depressed? If they have deep resentments, they will eventually show outwardly in the form of psychosomatic ills such as ulcers, severe headaches, arthritis, asthma, etc. This is not to imply that incorrect thinking is always the cause of any of the above illnesses, but in a large percentage of cases, negative thinking is the direct cause.

One woman had had a deep inward resentment for a number of years that was apparent to everyone except herself. It finally showed outwardly in the form of arthritis so severe that she was confined to a wheelchair. The strange thing was that although this was apparent to her family, she herself was completely unaware of the resentment. She had completely hidden it from herself and thought of herself as a very sweet and fair person.

Another student had developed tumors that were causing such pain that her doctor wanted to operate as soon as possible. She had been very resentful toward her husband for a number of years and had been guilty of much negative thinking. She could not see at first that she was at fault. When she finally understood that her own thinking may have caused her health problem, she made a remrkable about-face and disciplined herself to think positively in a very short period. At her next doctor's examination the tumors had disappeared. Her doctor thought he had made a mistake in his diagnosis.

These people looked and felt much older than their years because of their negative mental outlook. When they realized they could reverse not only their aging tendencies, but also their health problem, it was almost a miracle to them.

There is a strong influence that may affect even positive thinkers who do not indulge in resentful negative thinking to any great degree. Be aware of the power of the hypnotic effect of *false world concepts and beliefs* that have been around for so long that everyone accepts them as being true. You may ask, "How can you know that world beliefs are false when for hundreds of years these beliefs and concepts have been believed to be true?" Just because they have been believed for hundreds of years does not necessarily mean they are true. That is not a test of a true concept. The test is whether a belief has made the world a better place to live. If it has, then it is probably a true principle. Sadly, however, many of the world concepts have done nothing to help people, have not given them more food, a better standard of living, more education, or even any hope for the future.

One true test

There is only one true test by which world beliefs and concepts can be evaluated even if they have been believed for hundreds or thousands of years. That test is spoken of by a great teacher, who said, "By their fruits ye shall know them." So what are the fruits of the false world beliefs of the last thousand years?

One belief is the concept of aging. Age is a firm belief, therefore we have old age. There is a belief that "might makes right," therefore we have wars. There is a belief in power, therefore we have a few people always seeking to enslave millions of others.

These are the "fruits" of the past centuries of world beliefs and thinking! Can we really say these are correct and true? The answer is very obvious to most people. There is something wrong with these negative world beliefs and thinking, or we would have seen positive "fruits." The world would have been a better place to live by now, a "heaven on earth." But as of this moment, we certainly do not have a "heaven on earth," so we can safely assume that the majority of the negative world beliefs and concepts are not doing us any good.

So beware of the hypnotic effect of this wrong thinking. From this moment, let's protect ourselves from these false concepts and learn the truth about ourselves so the "truth can make us free."

How do we begin to do this? In chapter 4 you were given powerful words for you to say the moment you open your eyes each morning. This is a tool that will enable you to discipline your mind and neutralize this powerful universal influence. There are several other mind tools that will also accomplish this. The mind tools are exercises used to reach your subconscious level, where all of the erasing of false beliefs and attitudes and concepts must be done. We must throw out all of the "garbage" you were forced to believe. This "garbage" is now forcing you to grow old.

Your mind works in a very exact way. There are certain laws governing it just as there are laws of physics and mathematics. Two and two always equal four, never five. Laws also operate in the realm of the mind.

Set a goal

A mind tool used to execute the law of the mind that will trigger action almost immediately is that of setting a definite goal. In fact, that is the only way to trigger the subconscious mind. You must set a goal for yourself, and not only set it but *write it down*. This is a hard and fast rule. You do not have a goal unless it is written. It is not enough to say it or think it. The only way to trigger the mind is to write the goal down.

The goal we are striving for is that of youthful maturity, so that is what we shall write down. At the end of this chapter is a goal format. A hard and fast rule to be considered is that goals must be positive. Never write a negative goal such as "I don't want to grow old." This will only produce a negative effect in your subconscious mind. A much more positive statement is one like this: "I have youthful maturity with the energy and vitality of youth and the wisdom of maturity."

Notice the statement is made in the present tense. Your mind recognizes only the present, not the past or the future, so goals must always be stated in the present tense. If you write a statement such as "I will have youth," you are putting it in the future, and as far as your mind is concerned, it will always be in the future.

Goals should be made for three time periods: short-range goals, medium-range goals, and long-range goals. The short-range goal can be as short a time as one week to a month, the medium-range goal a year or two, and the long-range goal can be as far in the future as you wish. It does not matter if it is five years or twenty-five yars. What matters is that you are always reaching and striving toward your goal of youthful maturity. It really does not matter how long it takes you.

The goal of youthful maturity must be your goal alone. It cannot be your spouse's, your brother's or sister's, or anyone's except yours alone. If another person also wishes to make this a goal, this is fine. But you cannot force it upon anyone. You can change only yourself, never anyone else. Interestingly enough, when other people see how wonderful you look and feel, they become interested and also want to work toward this goal. But until that time, no matter how wonderful you think it would be for anyone else, remember they are free agents and can do as they want.

This is your goal format. Remember you do not have a goal until it is written down.

I, _____, now have as my goal *youthful maturity*. My first objective is to freeze my age where it is at the moment. Then I begin to reverse the process.

I have youthful maturity with the energy and vitality of youth and the wisdom of maturity.

On _____, I look and feel as I did three years ago. (If you were ill, or had a negative experience three years ago, use another year.)

On _____, I look and feel as I did six years ago.

On _____, I look and feel as I did ten, fifteen, twenty, ___, years ago.

(Cross out the numbers you do not want, leaving only the one you do want. If the year number is not listed, insert in the blank space the number you do want.)

Keep in mind that there is no way this cannot work. If on the date you have written down you do not have the desired result, simply put down another date and begin again. This is an individual matter; some people make rapid progress but others take longer. But it always works if you follow the correct sequence of steps. The only secret is *persistence*!

Let's attain the goal of youthful maturity using the building blocks of life!

CHAPTER 6

The Building Blocks
of Life

What are the building blocks of life: the crucial and yet surprisingly simple things most people fail to use? We have all learned about them in school, at home, in many magazines and thousands of books, but yet most of us totally ignore them.

Yes, that's right: good nutrition, wholesome foods, vitamins, minerals, etc. We all know about these things, but often we just try to stifle a yawn and go on to much more interesting subjects. We humans have a strange reaction to certain situations. If we are reasonably well, reasonably happy, and our problems are not too serious, we do nothing! We just float lazily on the surface of our conditions, with no direction in sight. It is not until problems or troubles become severe that we do anything at all.

How much better it would be if we would make the effort when all is well to raise to an optimum our health, happiness, and well-being! Strangely enough, most of us do not appreciate the magic in foods that are loaded with energy, vitality, and vigor until we have been ill and almost at death's door.

This is also true of the myth of old age. Until we begin to see the first signs of old age in the mirror, we almost totally ignore the things that would make age stop creeping up on us. Most of us keep our cars in much better shape than we do our bodies.

Vitamins and minerals necessary

In my opinion, a good vitamin-mineral supplement in addition to a healthful diet is very necessary because, among other things, our soil does not yield as much nutrition today as was the case fifty or even twenty-five years ago. Many other factors destroy the value of foods, such as overcooking, smoking, aspirin, diarrhea, and even excessive perspiration and stress. The list is endless.

Every day new discoveries are being made in the complex field of nutrition. One discovery recently made is that all vitamins, minerals, and enzymes interact with each other to produce changes in our bodies. All seem to have specific functions and each is dependent upon the others to carry out these specific functions. I find the simplest thing to do to make sure of having all the necessary ingredients of good body nutrition is to take a good brand of a *natural* vitamin-mineral supplement each day in addition to good wholesome food. Some people believe that a synthetic supplement is as good as a brand made from natural ingredients. However, because there are many things as yet undiscovered, most researchers will agree that there may be unknown "X" factors present in natural substances. Nature has been around longer than any one of us and had most things in almost a perfect balance until man tipped the balance in various ways.

Synthetic vitamins are made by reconstructing the molecular structure of a crystalline vitamin by chemically combining molecules from other sources. They have no synergists, enzymes, coenzymes, minerals, mineral activators, or coenzyme helpers. Therefore your body will get a smaller percentage of nutrition from synthetic vitamins than from the natural ones.

There are a few "power" foods that give you extra "mileage" from your calories, such as brewer's yeast, yogurt, lecithin, and sprouts, to name just a few. I have not always thought that it was important to be concerned about a nutritious diet, but through hard experiences of low vitality and illness and through the experiences of students, I now believe it is extremely important to learn to like such things. Brewer's yeast does not have as pleasant a taste as many foods do; however, the energy, vitality, and sense of well-being resulting from learning to like this drink make it well worth the effort. Even more important is the fact that these power foods actually help protect us from the effects of the ever-present bombardment of stress and tension in our society.

A breakfast drink

I have a very simple drink each morning in place of breakfast that gives me fifty times the amount of energy and well-being that bacon and eggs would give. It also has the added benefit of actually protecting me against stresses that I encounter each day. This is the recipe:

1. Combine 4 tablespoons of brewer's yeast with one 8-ounce glass of V-8 juice, tomato juice, grapefruit juice, or any acid base juice.

2. Add 2 tablespoons of lecithin and 1 tablespoon of wheat germ.

3. Blend in blender if you have one, or you can also make a paste and gradually stir in ingredients.

4. Add 2 or 3 ice cubes to chill.

This drink has very few calories so it has the added benefit of weight control.

One precaution, however: if you have never taken brewer's yeast, begin with only one teaspoon at first and gradually work to the four tablespoons in about thirty to sixty days. If you have never taken brewer's yeast, your body does not have the enzymes necessary to digest it, and needs time to develop the enzymes. If you do not take this precaution of beginning slowly, you may experience indigestion, bloating, and gaseous discomfort.

All of this is well worth the effort because even if you begin with only a teaspoon at first, within a few days you will experience a great energy uplift plus a relaxing effect at the same time. (The brewer's yeast spoken of here is not the fresh yeast used for baking.)

The wheat germ used in the drink contains vitamin E and is also an outstanding source of vitamin B_1. Tomato juice, grapefruit juice, or V-8 contain vitamin C. The lecithin is a fat emulsifier. So it is easy to see why this drink is such a "powerhouse" of energy. The

B-complex has long been known as an antistress factor as well as an energy-producing food.

One of my students made a similar drink using milk, which she said gave her the same effect. This is her recipe:

1. Combine 1 glass of cold skim milk with 4 tablespoons of brewer's yeast.

2. Add 2 tablespoons of lecithin and 1 tablespoon of wheat germ.

3. Add 2 packages of fructose (3 gm packets). Fructose is a natural sugar from fruits and vegetables and may be found in health food stores.

4. Add flavoring such as vanilla, or experiment with other flavors of pure extract, such as almond flavor, etc.

5. Add 2 tablespoons of oil, such as peanut, sesame, or safflower oil.

Blend in blender. Make it the night before and allow it to chill. If you do not like the acid-base juices, you may enjoy this drink.

No white sugar or flour

Train yourself to get rid of white sugar and white flour products. Both are "dead" foods. Even rats won't touch them. If you must have sweets, use honey, blackstrap molasses, pure maple syrup, fructose, or even date sugar. You need never eat another bit of white sugar for the rest of your life and your body will get from natural sources such as fruits or vegetables all of the sweets that are ncessary for health and, of course, youthful maturity.

Some of my students live in cold climates where fresh vegetables are difficult and expensive to obtain during the winter months. If this is also your problem, you can sprout seeds, such as alfalfa, bean sprouts, soybeans, etc. There are many many different kinds of seeds, all available in your local health food store. They are rich in the food nutrients our bodies need. For example, all sprouts contain vitamins A and B and in addition alfalfa sprouts are rich in vitamins D, E, B₂, K, and U (anti-ulcer vitamin). Soybeans and mung sprouts are also high in protein. When sprouted they can be used in salads or in place of salads, added to casseroles and soups, used in a sandwich in place of lettuce, used in Chinese dishes, etc. You can even add them to homemade rolls or bread. If you have too much for your use at any one time, they can be frozen or dried for future use because the nutrients in them are very stable and will not deteriorate rapidly. They will help your food budget as they are very inexpensive. Seeds are very simple to sprout and can be sprouted in a glass jar even if you live in a one-room apartment.

The wonderful egg

One of the best protein foods is the egg. Your body can assimilate more protein from eggs than from meat. Many times eggs are also a better buy at the market than meat, so again, your diet for "youthful maturity" need not be expensive. Begin to use more eggs in place of meat. If you use meat, the cheaper cuts of meat actually have more nutrition than the expensive cuts and it is simple to tenderize them with soy sauce, Worcestershire sauce, or even teriyaki sauce. On occasion, I have even tenderized pot roast with the juice left over from dill pickles. Any of the commercial tenderizers will also do the job of tenderizing the cheaper cuts of meat. Cheese is also an excellent source of protein and low-fat cottage cheese will give you a lot of nutrition at a cost low in both money and calories.

There is no one diet that is correct for everyone because each person is unique, not only in terms of food likes and dislikes, but also in beliefs about eating meat. This is an individual matter, but no matter what types of food you eat, the important thing is to follow the basic rules of proper nutrition. Your body needs fuel, and like your car, the better fuel mixture you provide for your nutritional needs, the better your body is going to react in terms of energy, vitality, looks, and, most important, the resistance to the "aging disease."

Building block foods

The building blocks you must have each day to reach your goal of youthful maturity no matter what your diet is are as follows:

1. Protein in the form of eggs or cheese, a good variety of protein vegetables, meat, seafood, or poultry.

To figure out individual protein requirements, simply divide the body weight by two and the result will indicate a very generous number of grams of protein, more than is actually required each day. For example, a person weighing 130 pounds would require at the most 65 grams of protein daily. If in doubt, eat a smaller amount, because latest research seems to indicate that a smaller amount is better than health authorities had formerly recommended. This appears to be true in achieving the goal of youthful maturity.

2. Fresh fruits (including citrus fruits) and vegetables should be eaten each day, not only for their vitamin and mineral content, but because your body must have enzymes each day to act as body catalysts. Enzymes are found in most fruits and vegetables, but are destroyed by heat. This is why it is so important to eat raw fruits and vegetables. An interesting test was done not too long ago on older people who were tired and showing their age with wrinkled skin and sagging of muscles. They were given enzymes each day and they soon experienced better health, more vitality, and a feeling of youthfulness.

3. Whole grain breads or cereals are necessary because these are muscle "fuels" that also aid in the digestion and assimilation of other foods. This type of carbohydrate is necessary to your body, but what is *not* necessary are the "junk food" carbohydrates such as french fries, doughnuts, or other sweets.

4. Some fats in the form of butter, margarine, or other table spread are also necessary because they are the carriers of the fat soluble vitamins A, D, E, and K. Fat also causes the release of a hormone, identified by H. W. Davenport as enterogastrone, which slows down the emptying time of the stomach, so hunger is not felt as quickly.

5. Milk should be included in the diet because it is

an excellent source of high-quality protein and phosphorus, plus calcium and riboflavin.

These are the basic building blocks for your body designed to give just ordinary energy, to keep you going at an average pace.

Power foods

The *power foods*, on the other hand, will give you super energy, super stamina, and super vitality. The power foods can help you actually freeze your age where you are now and slow down any future aging tendencies. The formula for reversing aging appearances is explained later. It is important to be familiar with the basic groundwork before going on to the super formula.

The following are the power foods that give you the most from your calories in terms of energy, vitality and well-being.

1. *Blackstrap molasses* contains a large amount of the B vitamins and is an unusually rich source of iron. It does have an unusual taste and you either like it or you don't. If you are one of those people who say "no" to blackstrap molasses, use instead the darkest unsulfured molasses you can find, or mix a little blackstrap molasses with your regular unsulfured kind. Molasses is made from the residue left from making sugar out of sugar cane or beets. The pure white "dead" sugar is sold as the premium product, whereas all the "goodies" are left in the residue. Many of our elders have allowed their blood to become anemic and weak. Blackstrap molasses will

build rich red youthful blood. It has twice as much iron as beef liver and is more easily digested. It may be stirred into milk, used with honey as a topping for pudding, mixed with yogurt, or even stirred in a cup of piping hot water as a healthful delicious coffee substitute (3 tablespoons to 1 cup of hot water).

2. *Yogurt* is another tremendous "power" food because it is an excellent source of easily assimilated high-quality protein plus calcium and riboflavin. It is excellent as a snack food because it is satisfying. It is advisable to buy the unflavored kind and mix in your own fresh or frozen fruit. You may mash a banana and stir it in, or mix in applesauce or fresh or frozen strawberries.Or you may buy it in a health food store because in too many instances the commercial yogurt purchased in a grocery store contains "fillers" and white sugar. In any case, read the label as this is now the only consumers' protection.

Yogurt is especially helpful in counteracting the "age syndrome" because many people have had a decline in the secretion of hydrochloric acid, an enzyme needed for digestive vigor. Yogurt helps to stimulate the production of this enzyme and this in turn helps bring about a more youthful digestive ability because of the beneficial changes in the physical condition of the bowels.

3. *Wheat germ* is worth its weight in gold as an outstanding source of vitamins B_1 and E. It can be mixed with other foods such as meat loaf, used as coating for broiled fish or chicken, or sprinkled over salads. Several experiments have been done with older people using wheat germ oil. One group each received 1½ teaspoons of wheat germ oil daily to take

internally and to use as a moisturizer for the face. Wheat germ oil softens and acts as a barrier to keep the water in the skin instead of allowing it to evaporate. Within a short time a large percentage of these people had reversed their age characteristics from ten to fifteen years. The vitamin E in the wheat germ has many other beneficial effects on the body, which will be discussed in detail later.

4. *Lecithin* takes its place among our power foods because it helps to rebuild cells or organs that need rebuilding. It reduces the cholesterol level in the blood. It prevents that drawn look while losing weight because it redistributes the weight from where you don't want it to where you do want it. It has also been found to be a brain food. Science has proved that lecithin is a substance in the brain tissue associated with retention of information.

It is also a powerful instrument for keeping the aging process at bay because it fills out and softens aging skin. In many older people it produces great alertness.

Lecithin can be easily sprinkled over salads or cereals or stirred into drinks or even gravies because it is almost tasteless. A very tasty table spread can be made by blending 1 cup of butter and 1 tablespoon powdered lecithin with 1 cup of safflower oil.

5. *Liver* is also one of the super foods of all times. Dr. Benjamin Ershoff of the Nutritional Research Institute found that liver is one of the most marvelous foods for enhancing the ability to resist stress. It is an incredibly rich source of vitamins, minerals, and protein. A three-ounce serving of beef liver has more vitamin A than carrots, and more thiamine-niacin-

vitamin C, iron, phosphorus, potassium, copper, and zinc than most foods. However, the real secret to liver's antistress action seems to be contained in its complex of enzymes and metabolites.

Although many people do not enjoy the taste of liver, this is no excuse because it can be included in the diet in the form of desiccated, or dried, liver, which has had much of the fat and tissue removed. This is truly a super energy food for the youthful maturity energy diet.

6. *Brewer's yeast* is also an incredible form of super energy. This power food has 16 different vitamins including all of the B complex, 16 amino acids, and 14 minerals, including the trace minerals that are so essential. It also has 36 percent protein (sirloin steak has only 23 percent).

Research done by Dr. Tom Spies of Birmingham, Alabama, should convince anyone who wishes to "turn off their age" that this is a food worth learning to like. He gave 893 men and women who both looked old and felt old large amounts of brewer's yeast and other nutritional supplements. In a few months an astonishing change took place in these people. Gone were the weakness, lethargy, depression, and exhaustion. In their place were cheerfulness, optimism, a sense of well-being, and a remarkable increase in physical and mental stamina; and the majority of the people began to look younger and fresher. Their skin developed a lustre and healthful texture where before it had been dry and wrinkled. There was a sparkle in their eyes and their physical movements were vigorous and youthful.

Dr. K. Sugiura at the Sloan-Kettering Institute for

Cancer Research found that brewer's yeast seemed to protect rats from getting cancer although they had been fed cancer-causing ingredients in their diets. The control group all suffered from cancer nodules of the liver induced by the diet.

We have also had excellent results in our classes when students began to eat these power foods and of course followed the rest of the program. One remarkable case was a couple 73 and 83 years of age. When they began the program both were very tired, had no interest in life, and just seemed to shuffle along. They could not remember many simple things. Within three months they were walking very energetically, their memories improved, and they again had a great interest in life. Each seemed to drop from ten to fifteen years off their age.

These are the "power" foods that will provide a rich fuel mixture for your body. They will pay off for you in terms of energy, vitality, and health, plus the added bonus of being able to turn off your age.

Some people have been placed on a salt-free diet by their doctors. For those people, I'd like to pass on what many students did. They began to substitute kelp for salt because it has a tangy salty taste, yet is all natural with many minerals and can easily be used as a salt substitute.

Vitamins

What part do vitamins play in this "no aging" game? Since vitamins are active members of an organization of nutrients that work closely together to keep your body working as it should, they become vitally important. Without vitamins you could not use the food you eat, children would stop growing, and young adults would be old at age 25. But before any of this would happen, you'd be a suffering, tired-out human being. It has only been in the last few years that vitamins have been known to be as important as they really are. Foods used to be full of good vitamins and minerals. Lately, because of all the preservatives, additives, soil depletion, and synthetic products, vitamins are not as plentiful in our foods. We now have to make a special effort to get them even for normal purposes, let alone such an important undertaking as turning off your age. You should be taking a natural, all-purpose vitamin-mineral supplement and not just one or two vitamins alone. Vitamins and minerals are linked together as intricately as a very fine chain. If one link is missing, the whole chain will be broken.

It is not necessary to list all the vitamins because many wonderful health books can give you that information, but the ones that are vital in helping you turn off your age are the vitamin B-complex, vitamin C and vitamin E. Minerals are also very important because without minerals the vitamins cannot function. So to be on the safe side, get a very good brand of a natural vitamin-mineral product.

If you are serious about turning off your age, you must train yourself to eat the marvelous energy-packed "power" foods. These foods have the ability to help you retain your youthful maturity indefinitely. So go to your favorite health food store and load up on these "jet fuels" for your body.

As you begin to learn about a few basic body nutrients, it is surprising how simple it becomes to put together a very tasty, inexpensive, nutritious meal. Your body is not demanding, but it does enjoy having premium foods instead of the empty calories most of us have been used to eating. It will show its appreciation to you in the form of healthful, radiant looks, tremendous energy, vitality, and last, but most important, youthful maturity for many, many years. You will then see in the mirror the beautiful total person you really are!

CHAPTER 7

High Energy Is Yours

High energy is a by-product of a diet aimed at turning off your age. You will be both surprised and delighted at your tremendous energy level as you continue your "de-aging" diet. This feeling of well-being and high energy will be one of the first rewards that will make you want to continue this new way of life. The energy lift in itself is worth the small effort necessary to change your eating habits.

There have been many diets aimed at giving you what you most desire, youthful maturity. Millions of words have been written on what kinds of foods will help you to feel your best. Presented in this chapter are those I consider most desirable as well as the research that has been done to show the greater effectiveness of some food over others. Research scientists are discovering more and more about how nutrition relates not only to the aging process, but all health-related problems. As one research scientist on aging put it:

Your body is very much like a car. When it's new there are few problems, but as the car gets older small things begin to go wrong at first, such as loss of good gas mileage. Perhaps it does not start as easily on cold mornings, or there is a knock in the motor you have not heard before, or there is not as much power as before. You can go to a garage and get these minor things taken care of, but from that time on you must pay close attention to keeping the car in tip-top shape. You cannot afford to put off changing the oil or getting a tune-up because as the car gets older the various systems begin to wear out if they are not taken care of immediately. Our bodies are just like that. Several systems begin to slow down and each system is dependent upon the other. It then becomes very important to pay attention to the various needs of each system.

You must begin to pay attention to the nutritional needs of your body. You must begin to pay attention to the motor requirements of your body, and exercise to keep the parts and joints moving smoothly. You must also begin to pay attention to mental requirements, such as new interests to keep your mind active and curious.

The influence of diets

One of the first reports on the nutritional importance of diets in relation to aging came from Alfred McCann in his book, *The Science of Keeping Young,* where he stated that it is possible to take two animals that came from the same litter and produce vitality, energy, and robust health in one and signs of old age in the other by merely changing their diet. Dr. Clive McCay reported in "Nutritional Experiments on Longevity" *(Journal of American Geriatrics Society* 6, No. 3, March 1958): "Thirty years ago we became convinced that the disease of old age in experimental animals such as white rats could be changed by control of the diet. We know that the most effective control of the diseases of later life must begin early, but that the latter half of life may be influenced even when dietary changes are introduced in middle life." This is a very conservative statement because now with much later research we know that dietary changes in middle life and even beyond have a very great influence upon the aging process.

There have been other experiments dealing with the multiplication of the cells for an indefinite time. Dr. Alexis Carrel, a noted cell biologist in the early part of the century, achieved fame for his experiment in growing chicken cells in tissue culture under ideal conditions. He reported they could be maintained and be kept multiplying as long as conditions were favorable. Several other laboratories using Carrel's techniques confirmed these results. Thus for a long time it was believed that the cell itself could live and divide indefinitely were it not confined to a body and thus subject to other weakening factors such as infections, pollution, free radicals, etc. However, recent research has not confirmed these earlier experiments. Repeated attempts to culture cells indefinitely have failed. Why the experiments now fail no one knows.

Causes of aging

Dr. Leonard Hayflick, who has done much research at Stanford University on the process of aging, believes that there are a number of "physiological decrements" that occur in nondividing cells such as the brain and muscle cells, which correlate with the aging process. They include decreased DNA and RNA synthesis. DNA (deoxyribonucleic acid) and RNA (ribonucleic acid) are two main forms of nucleic acid.

Other scientists believe that aging is caused by process of oxidation and through free radicals. A free radical is a wild molecule with a lot of energy and a missing electron. It causes a lot of destruction by reacting promiscuously with other molecules, influencing them to also become free radicals. It can be likened to a mad dog running completely out of control along the street, biting other animals in his path, causing them all to also become mad. Free radicals enter our bodies most of the time from foods that have been oxidized by X rays, cosmic rays, pollution, and nuclear fallout. When they enter the body they damage DNA cells as well as many other cell structures. DNA is the blueprint that leads cells to divide in a perfect replica of the first cell, which they do in all young bodies. After years of exposure to free radicals and oxidation, which destroy the perfect blueprint, the cells begin to divide in misshaped forms, thus causing the appearance of aging. (Do not despair, as this can be counteracted by correct nutrients.)

Another interesting research project on aging is the linkage theory, which proposes that protein molecules become linked with other protein molecules. When these doubled or tripled molecules happen, it is as if the cell has been "gummed up."

The most recent theory of aging concerns the outer surface of the cell. On the outer surface of each cell are so-called "antennae," which do for the cell what an antenna does for a television set. When these "antennae" are damaged, the cell is unable to pull in a "clear picture" and the aging process begins.

Dr. Alex Comfort, director of the Gerontology Research Group of the University College in London, said the goal of anti-aging research follows a number of lines of attack. Some of these include the study of why the metabolic processes change and the immune mechanisms go wrong with age. Dr. Robert Zellis, associate professor of medicine at the University of California, advocates using proteins that have a lower content of saturated fats, such as chicken, turkey, veal, and fish instead of beef, lamb, or pork. He advises that if you choose the latter to be sure to trim off all fat before cooking and also to pour off all grease that cooks out of the meat.

First-class proteins are very important to maintain youthful maturity. A team of five researchers in the Department of Nutrition and Food Science and Clinical Research Center of MIT have measured the rate of protein synthesis from newborn infants to the elderly. They found that a baby synthesized 17.4 grams of protein, but the rate dropped all the way to 1.9 percent in the elderly. This means that a baby's body was able to use 17.4 percent of all protein it was fed, while an elderly person's body was able to utilize only 1.9 percent of the protein although the quality and amount of protein was equally as good as the baby's.

First-class protein needed

What does this mean in terms of "turning off your age"? We certainly cannot eat that much more protein to allow our body to make up the difference. No, what it does mean is that we must be much more selective about the quality of our protein. It must be first-class protein at all times. The diets of the Hunzas, Vilcabambans, and long-lived Soviets are geared to enable their bodies to utilize a much higher percentage of protein than ours do. Their protein needs of their bodies are satisfied with only 35 to 50 grams a day, compared with North Americans, who eat more than 100 grams daily. Their bodies seem to utilize the smaller amounts better than ours do our larger amounts. However, our eating habits are totally different. The Pakistani Hunzas begin the day with tea flavored with milk, and—surprisingly—salt. The Vilcabambans eat much cereals and grains, while the Soviet Caucasus begin the day with sour milk, cheese, and yogurt.

Dr. Ronald E. Gots, director of the National Medical Advisory Service, published a sample menu based on the diets of these long-living people, but modified to agree with our food habits. He suggests the following breakfast:

½ cup plain yogurt with 1 medium banana sliced in the yogurt

2 slices whole-wheat toast with 2 ounces cottage cheese

1 tablespoon cherry jelly

Coffee or tea

Dr. Frank's diet

Although these sample anti-aging diets are all helpful, by far the best one in my judgment is that of

Dr. Benjamin Frank of New York City. His records are bulging with records of patients helped for the past twenty years by his diet approach. His diet seems to neutralize all of the theoretical damage done by free radicals, linkage, cell multiplication failure of RNA and DNA, etc. His own theory is that there is a "loss of energy in the cell," caused by years of exposure to pollution, radiation, poor nutrition, lack of exercise, etc.

He believes that the answer to the aging process is to eat foods high in nucleic acids, such as sardines, as well as other fish. Muscle meats such as steaks, chops, and roasts, and dairy fats should not be eaten more than once a week. Liver should be eaten once a week, but during the balance of the week, seafoods, particularly sardines, should be eaten. Avoid canned foods and eat fresh fruits and vegetables instead. Try to find organically grown fruits and vegetables because chemical fertilizers deplete the soil of trace minerals. Cut out sugar and starches entirely or to a minimum. If you do not eat any white sugar or white flour the rest of your life your body would be much better off. Instead substitute honey, blackstrap molasses, or fructose for white sugar.

Use salt and strong seasonings sparingly, substituting herbs instead. It is very important to drink at least four glasses of water daily, as well as two glasses of skimmed milk and one glass of vegetable juice. (This will keep uric acid from forming in your body.)

The vegetable juice should be prepared fresh daily using a juicer. Mix from 1 teaspoon to as much as 3 tablespoons of brewer's yeast in the juice. If you have never used brewer's yeast, remember the advice given in chapter 6 to work up to the 3 tablespoons very slowly as your body does not have the enzymes necessary to digest the yeast. When you drink your skimmed milk, add ½ to 1 tablespoon of acidophilus powder as this helps to maintain favorable intestinal flora.

Eat one egg daily, preferably purchased in a health food store because these eggs come from chickens fed natural grains and allowed to scratch food from the ground. You may also eat low-calorie cottage cheese. If you are overweight, do not eat any hard cheeses until you have your desired weight. Always eat whole grain bread, never white bread, even the enriched kind. The so-called enriched white bread has had 17 important nutrients removed and 5 synthetic nutrients added and it is then labeled "enriched." Sprouted bread and breads made with several different grains are excellent. Read the label to make sure there is no sugar added.

Once or twice a week eat one or more of the following cooked fresh vegetables: peas, lima beans, soybeans, or lentils. Each day, in addition to a fresh vegetable salad, eat one of these vegetables: asparagus, radishes, mushrooms, spinach, cauliflower, or celery. (They can be added to your salad.)

It is important to supplement your diet with vitamins and minerals. It is impossible to eat enough to give our bodies the proper nutrition in these days of "foodless" foods unless you also include good vitamin-mineral supplements. These should include vitamin C (with bioflanoids), vitamin E, the complete vitamin B complex, cod-liver oil, RNA-DNA tablets, bonemeal and a good complete product containing minerals. All of these can be purchased in health food stores.

Garlic and onions have been found to contain much of the nutrients we lack in our ordinary diet. When you make a salad, always add an onion. Garlic becomes a little touchy in our society, but it is possible to purchase garlic capsules that you can take without the unpleasant side effect of the garlic odor.

It is also important to include in your anti-aging diet at least 2 to 3 tablespoons of lecithin daily, which can be sprinkled on your salad, added to soups, etc. Wheat germ is also a very valuable nutrient. It can be used to add to meat loaf, or instead of bread crumbs if you are breading anything. It can also be stirred into juices.

As you can see, this diet is very rich in nucleic acids plus fluids and vitamin-minerals. The nucleic acids are spread in foods throughout the week, so you will have an intake of one or two grams daily.

(Of course if you are under a physician's care—as you should be if you have any kind of medical problem—and have another diet, always check with him first as he certainly knows your condition better than anyone else.)

In Dr. Frank's words, "This diet is perfectly safe and has proved effective in slowing down the aging process and returning many who were seriously sick to good health." This is really an understatement, as many of Dr. Frank's patients have not only slowed the aging process but even reversed the aging tendencies by ten to twenty years. This has been both in appearance, and in high energy and vitality.

CHAPTER 8

Muscle Tone
through
Body Movements

Muscles must be kept in action if you are to turn off your age. If you are not active, very shortly there will be a gradual slowdown and deterioration of your body movements. Everyone has seen the slow shuffle of very old people, head and shoulders bent, unable even to raise their head anymore. The dangerous aspect of this gradual slowdown is that it is not noticed by the individual and many times not even by the people that see them every day. Sadly, if an occurrence is not shocking or sudden, it is often acceptable.

Allowing yourself to slow down unnecessarily is the very saddest fact of all. Nature has given us an ever-renewing machine if we keep the hinges and joints lubricated and the parts moving quietly and smoothly.

Exercise doesn't have to be dull

Many students in our "Turn Off Your Age" classes moan when exercise is mentioned. However, it is not necessary to do dull sit-ups or push-ups. Surprisingly, you need not even do exercise every day. Research has shown that if you do exercises three times a week that will force each muscle to two-thirds of its maximum holding power, that is quite sufficient to keep the muscles in optimum tone.

So many different kind of exercises have been developed that there is no excuse for anyone not to do something to tone up muscles. One of the best exercises is the body stretch. Muscles in action stretch, contract, and relax. The blood vessels within also stretch, contract, and relax in turn. When you are stimulated internally and quickened through proper body movement, good circulation is created and your entire body benefits. When the correct body movements are done, it creates pulsations and concentrations in the tissues that come across as feelings of good muscle tone. Firm muscle tone creates a great feeling of being alive, of having strength and vigor to do things for long periods without tiring. Good muscle tone gives firmness and slender lines to the body. Begin to practice stretching your body each day. When you first wake up while lying in your bed is a very good time to do this.

Are you out of shape?

Below are a few questions that will give you a hint of where you're at in this business of keeping your body parts moving smoothly.

1. Are you out of breath after climbing ten steps?

2. Have you found it difficult to stay alert during a lecture or class even when you have had eight to ten hours of sleep the night before?

3. Have you ever gone shopping and had to sit and rest after just a short time?

If you answered "yes" to even one of these questions, chances are that you have not concerned yourself with the importance of physical fitness.

In our classroom work, it is the exceptional student that has any kind of an exercise program at all. Most of the students will say, "Oh, I get enough exercise around the house, shopping or gardening." But that will not do because there are several types of exercises and any one of those activities will not exercise your entire body. Exercise directly affects your whole body. It helps lose weight, gives you greater physical strength and endurance, relieves tension, and improves appearance. It even stimulates mental activity and keeps you looking and feeling younger.

A student who looked much older than her 35 years had just exactly that experience. When she came to class she was twenty pounds overweight, uninterested in life in general, and came only because her husband had threatened divorce if she did not do something. She decided to jog simply because she lived close to her son's school and they had a professional jogging track. Her son joined her each morning so it became an enjoyable treat for her. She did nothing else in the program except the jogging. She did not follow any particular health program, did not change her diet, but at the end of three months she had already lost fifteen pounds, was alive and vital once more, and was very much interested in things around her.

Another student also chose jogging for her exercise. She was 65 when she joined the class and had not done any type of exercise prior to this time. She began very slowly at first, but at the end of several months was able to jog one mile. She also looked and felt much better because she had an interest in life once more. The most astounding thing about this student was that after several years of jogging, she decided to enter a marathon race, won it and made the headlines. Now, ten years later, she's won about eight or nine races and each time makes the papers because women, or men for that matter, are not supposed to win marathon races at 75 years of age.

In choosing jogging for their exercises, these students were doing an aerobic exercise. Aerobic exercises demand oxygen, but do not create as great an oxygen debt as an anaerobic exercise such as high-speed running or swimming or weight training.

Four types of exercise

There are four basic types of exercises and you must decide which type will best suit your body needs.

1. The *aerobic* exercises are best for a person who has not exercised in a long time to begin with, because they can be continued for a long period of time and produce a good training effect on the lungs, heart, and overall circulatory and respiratory systems. Some of these exercises include walking, hiking,

cycling, rope jumping, handball, tennis, and similar activities.

2. The *isotonic* exercises involve muscle concentration that develop muscle tone, strength, endurance power, flexibility, balance, agility, and coordination. Examples of this type of exercise include weight lifting and calisthenic exercises.

3. *Isometric* exercises also develop muscle tone, size, strength, and power, but the blood flow through the muscle tissues is constricted during an isometric exercise so there is little effect on general endurance. Examples of this type of exercise include tightening the fist, flexing the biceps, pressing the palms together, or pushing against an immovable object such as a wall. An exercise that is marvelous for developing the bust for women is this: simply push the palms of your hands together when your arms are out from your body and level with your bustline. Do this about fifteen to twenty times each day and in a very short time the bust muscles will be toned up and you will be able to see the difference.

4. *Anaerobic* exercises are from both the isometric and isotonic, but their purposes differ. These exercises are used to build up speed, power, and muscular strength. They require so much oxygen that they can be continued for only a short period. Running, both short and long distance; swimming, weight training, and heavy calisthenics or gymnastics are examples of these exercises.

The best exercise program is one that develops overall fitness. You should include warm-up exercises followed by a series of conditioning exercises and then a sport you enjoy, such as swimming, tennis, jogging, cycling, etc.

I have never enjoyed doing exercises until I discovered that dancing is a marvelous exercise. Always do something you really enjoy doing; then it is a positive activity for you and not something you think you must do.

Don't get discouraged

The most important thing to remember when developing a serious exercise program is not to get discouraged. Many people have not done serious body movements since high school. It will take at least twenty-one days to form a habit for exercise. So just *persist* and don't be too hard on yourself when the program does not go as smoothly as you had imagined.

A few students in our Turn Off Your Age classes have wondered if the people who live well into the 90s or even over 100 have an exercise program. We find that most of these people usually did such things as gardening, jogging, walking, or similar forms of exercise as a way of life, not as a separate exercise program.

Dr. Gabe Mirkin of the University of Maryland has found out many interesting and positive things that exercise will do for you, including improvement of a person's sexual performance. He also feels that the most important exercises are those that train your heart, such as running, jogging, ice skating, roller skating, bicycling, jumping rope, and cross-country skiing. He says that if you cannot get outside you can do them indoors on a stationary bicycle, and also do your jogging on a treadmill. The bad thing about such stationary exercises is that they can get boring, and you should enjoy exercising.

Dr. Mirkin wrote that the most important thing about training your heart is to bring your heartbeat up to about 120 beats a minute. However, he also warns that anyone over 35 who has not exercised should first get a stress electrocardiogram to find out how his or her heart will behave with virgorous exercise. Have your doctor measure your heart while you exercise and he will tell you the maximum pulse rate that is safe for you.

Even a little is better than none

Perhaps you think you do not have the time to exercise as much as you would like. Many people feel that if you can't do it right, you should not try at all. However, in the case of exercise even a little bit is better than none at all. Any exercise is worthwhile, and if you have not exercised for years, start at a level you can maintain and try to increase. There are three warning signs that you are overdoing it with your exercising. They are chest pains during exercise, heart palpitations when you are idle, and unexplained dizziness. If you have any of these symptoms, stop exercising and check with your doctor.

An interesting case involving jogging is in the files of the President's Physical Fitness Council. A Texas physician reported that one of his patients was so depressed after several heart attacks that he resolved to kill himself. To spare his wife he decided to make his death seem accidental, so he took up jogging in the hope that he would literally run himself into the ground. "Sure enough," reported the doctor, "he collapsed on the first try, but he didn't die, so the next day he tried again. In fact he kept trying to kill himself by jogging for a whole week. But by the end of the first week, he was feeling better. Soon he felt so much stronger and happier that he decided to live." Psychiatrists have found that exercise—but not so extreme!—can rid mentally ill patients of anxieties and drive away depression.

Three exercises for quick results

The three exercises that I think are the easiest for most of us to do and seem to show the quickest results in the shortest time with the least amount of money spent are:

1. Aerobic dancing, which is especially recommended to tired housewives. This type of dancing includes high-kick dancing done to music. It also includes "disco" dancing or any dancing done in your own home to music that will encourage you to dance for at least fifteen minutes and raise your heart beat to 120 if you are 45 or younger. If you are over that age, raise it to from 119 to 100, depending on your age. In other words, the older you are, the less your heart rate should be raised. If you are 70 or over, do not raise it over 100 unless you have been exercising all of your life, or unless you have checked with your doctor. However, do not be too hesitant in this matter of exercise. Dr. Perola Ostrand, a Swedish exercise-physiologist, says, "As a general rule, moderate activity is less harmful to the healthy person than inactivity."

2. Jogging is also very beneficial to most people, men or women. You need only wear comfortable loose-fitting clothes, but you do need to have good running shoes. Do not run on cement. Run on a jogging track, dirt, or grass. Begin slowly by walking first for a few days if you are not used to exercise. Then run just about one-half block and gradually lengthen the jogging time. Alternate the jogging and the walking when you begin to feel tired. However, you must either walk or jog for at least twenty minutes or it will not do you much good. At the end of the first week, you will notice how much better you will feel, both mentally and physically.

3. The third type of exercise that I personally feel is most helpful is jumping rope. Jumping rope for 15 minutes each day reduces the thighs, hips, and buttocks. These bulges and spreads are the hardest for women to trim. Again, if you have not exercised for a long time, do begin slowly. Five minutes of jumping rope is equivalent of a set of tennis or nine holes of golf. The wonderful thing about jumping rope is that you can jump anywhere. You can jump in a space as small as a closet, or by your desk in your office, in the kitchen—any place that is convenient. Women should always wear a bra for support when jumping rope. When you jump, you must land on the balls of your feet. Turn on some music, time yourself, and jump to music. At first begin with only ten counts and add just two or three each day until you have worked up to either 200 counts or have jumped for 15 minutes, whichever is longer.

Follow these tips when jumping:

1. Work your rope from your wrists because too much arm action will make you too tired too fast.

2. Jump very lightly, like a leaf floating to the ground and always come down on the balls (front) of your feet.

3. Breathe through your nose.

4. Don't look at the rope, look straight ahead.

5. If you have a mirror, jump in front of it and you will be able to check your muscle reactions.

6. If you get tired, you may stop, but you must bend over then and stretch your body. Touch your toes and inhale. Put your hands on the floor and breathe in through the nose and out through the mouth. Do a low stretch and stay there until you feel rested. Then begin jumping again.

7. Always time yourself so you will get at least fifteen minutes after you have worked up to that time.

Take your pulse

Learn to take your pulse and you can determine how much exercise you need. Place your hand over your heart or find your pulse beat in either of your large arteries at the sides of your neck. With the right thumb on the chin, the fingers can easily feel the artery in front of the muscle running down the side of the neck.

After you have found your pulse, count it *accurately* for six seconds. Begin by counting your pulse when at rest. Count it for exactly six seconds, add a zero on the end of the number, and that is your resting pulse. After exercising vigorously for fifteen minutes, assuming reasonably good health, again take your pulse and it should be from 100 to 120 counts, depending on your age. If it is more than that, slow down your exercise.

You must exercise at least three times a week with no more than two days lapsing between workouts or you will forfeit any gains. You can reach your optimal state of fitness in three to six months. Once you attain it, you must maintain it by regular workouts. If you discontinue your exercising, you will completely lose all gains in five weeks.

You may be like one of our early students who hated the thought of exercise, but agreed to try it at least for the duration of the class. At the end of that period, she'd lost twenty pounds, looked ten years younger, and felt twenty-five years younger. She said she'd never give it up, that it was her "youth pill." Life was very enjoyable for her, whereas before she'd dreaded the thought of getting out of bed to another boring day.

On the next page is a cardiovascular fitness record for a jump-roping program. You can take your pulse and record it and observe your progress. Your recovery time should be just a few minutes after you take your pulse after active exercise. In other words, take your pulse the moment you stop exercising and record it. Wait about five minutes, take it again and it should be back to the resting pulse, or very close at least.

Do not allow yourself to slow down when it is not necessary. However, you and you alone are the only one who can make it happen. So go for it!

Cardiovascular Fitness Record
Skip Ropeing Program

Date:

Name:

Week	Day	Duration in Minutes	Rest Pulse Rate	Active Pulse Rate	Recovery Pulse Rate	Points	Total
1	M						
	T						
	W						
	T						
	F						
	S						
2	M						
	T						
	W						
	T						
	F						
	S						
3	M						
	T						
	W						
	T						
	F						
	S						
4	M						
	T						
	W						
	T						
	F						
	S						
5	M						
	T						
	W						
	T						
	F						
	S						
6	M						
	T						
	W						
	T						
	F						
	S						

NOTE: Skip at a frequency of 70-80 steps per minute.

Week	Day	Duration in Minutes	Rest Pulse Rate	Active Pulse Rate	Recovery Pulse Rate	Points	Total
7	M						
	T						
	W						
	T						
	F						
	S						
8	M						
	T						
	W						
	T						
	F						
	S						
9	M						
	T						
	W						
	T						
	F						
	S						
10	M						
	T						
	W						
	T						
	F						
	S						
11	M						
	T						
	W						
	T						
	F						
	S						
12	M						
	T						
	W						
	T						
	F						
	S						

Week	Day	Duration in Minutes	Rest Pulse Rate	Active Pulse Rate	Recovery Pulse Rate	Points	Total
13	M						
	T						
	W						
	T						
	F						
	S						
14	M						
	T						
	W						
	T						
	F						
	S						
15	M						
	T						
	W						
	T						
	F						
	S						
16	M						
	T						
	W						
	T						
	F						
	S						
17	M						
	T						
	W						
	T						
	F						
	S						
18	M						
	T						
	W						
	T						
	F						
	S						

CHAPTER 9

Mirror Image Technique

One of the great master secrets of the world, which very few people know, is that your subconscious mind does not know the difference between a real and an imagined experience. Startling, isn't it? Your subconscious mind cannot tell the difference between something that is happening externally and something that is being imagined internally. Knowledge of this simple fact can enable anyone to trigger his or her subconscious mind in any direction, reach any goal, achieve any dream. This is a law of the mind and always works if you use it correctly.

The technique utilizing this law has been used in many sports. Well-known golfers have used the technique of imagery to teach people to play superb golf. Skiers have been taught to parallel down a steep slope totally relaxed and in perfect form. Using this method, swimmers are taught dry land swimming before going into the water. When they are in the water their subconscious mind takes over and, surprisingly, they can swim perfectly without effort the very first time. A few years ago, basketball players in a famous university were divided into two groups. One group practiced shooting baskets on the gymnasium floor. The other group did not go near the gym, but sat in the classroom and practiced seeing themselves throwing the ball into the air and hitting the basket every time. At the end of a month the group that had been physically practicing in the gym had improved 18 percent and the group using mental imagery had improved 19 percent. Research has proved that whenever anyone imagines themselves throwing a ball and hitting the basket as these players did, the muscles that are involved give a slight twitch, so slight that if electrodes were not fastened on the muscles it would not be noticeable.

Many people find this easy to believe in the field of sports or simple things, but find it harder to believe in an area such as turning off your age. However, it does not matter if you do not believe this technique will work. If you do it even with unbelief, in time your mind will accept it and you will then believe.

Always keep in mind that you are a total person and must work in all areas—the physical area, using diet and exercise, and the mental area, using the mirror imagine technique and mental imagery, and remember at all times that in the spiritual area you are much, much greater than you think you are.

Your subconscious mind functions in an automatic way. Even though at first you may not believe the technique will work, if you persist, in a short time your mind will accept it and you will believe it. With some students it is as short a time as twenty-one days, with others it is somewhat longer.

Disbelief into belief

Your mind will form a habit if you persist, even if you do not believe at first. You may have a great big "disbelief" at first but as you persist that disbelief will grow smaller and smaller each time you practice both the mirror image technique and mental imagery until you reach the "point of change." At this point the mind begins to turn itself around and you will begin to have thoughts such as, "Well, maybe I really can turn off my age," or "Maybe I really can like myself unconditionally." Each day as you practice the technique, the disbelief gets smaller and smaller until one day you get a small "belief." This tiny "belief" keeps growing and growing until one wonderful day you wake up in the morning with the marvelous feeling of realization that you have formed a habit of positive belief. At that time your mind will begin to turn around all of your physical bodily functions that have been leading you toward old age. Now your mind will first begin to "turn off your age," and then gradually begin to reverse your aging tendencies. The only secret to this is to keep *persisting*, no matter what happens, or even if you get discouraged. Just keep trying!

There are two steps to the mirror image technique. The first step in this process is doing the mirror exercise, a very simple but effective exercise. You may be tempted to believe that because of its very simplicity it cannot possibly work. Please do not be misled into this kind of irrational thinking. We have proved with thousands of students that it is at this point the change must begin, regardless of past negative experiences. Before there can be improvement in any area of your life you *must* accept yourself right as you are at this moment. If you cannot do this, you will make only very temporary progress.

Accept yourself as you are

Keep in mind that no matter what your past has been, even if it has been the most negative living, the most overwhelming, terrible mistakes, or even great problems, it does not matter! Realize you did the best you could at the time with the knowledge and childhood conditioning you had. Every person always does the best he can, even if he makes mistake after mistake. *At that time* it is the best he can do.

So right now at this point, accept yourself as you are and then let's go on to greater and greater possibilities. As an example of this, one of our students had been an abused child. Unfortunately, this type of training in early childhood perpetuates itself, so her children were also abused children. She blamed and condemned herself so bitterly that it seemed almost impossible to overcome this negative experience in her life. However, she employed the mirror technique, even though at first she did not believe anything positive would happen. She accepted herself in spite of all the mistakes she'd made and inflicted upon others. Eventually she realized she could have done nothing else because of her earlier false training. She forgave herself and accepted herself right where she was. Then a miracle happened. In forgiving herself, she was able to completely change her behavior toward her children and became as wonderful a mother as she'd been abusive in the past.

The mirror technique

The mirror technique is practiced as follows:

1. Upon arising in the morning, before combing your hair, shaving, putting on makeup, etc., go to your mirror, look yourself directly in the eye, and say (out loud if possible), with as much emotion as you can, "*I like myself* **unconditionally**." If you are in a situation that you cannot say it out loud, at least mouth the words to yourself. There will be at least a moment or two during the day when you will be alone, and at that time look in the mirror and repeat the statement out loud.

2. The last thing at night before going to bed, repeat this exercise, again looking yourself in the mirror and saying to yourself, "*I like myself* **unconditionally**." The key word here is *unconditionally*. It means you accept yourself without any conditions. All of our lives we have been putting conditions on our ability to like ourselves. Thoughts such as these usually run through the mind: "Oh, yes I can like myself if I lose twenty pounds, or if I stop smoking, or if I control my temper, etc." Always these negative statements seem to control the thinking process. But now it becomes very important to erase the conditions and accept yourself just where you are at this moment.

Your reactions at first may be rather odd. You will certainly get an uncomfortable feeling inside you. You may laugh heartily or you may even cry. One student began to cry each time he said, "I like myself unconditionally," because in his childhood he had been so rejected, so lonely, that he did not believe anyone could like him. He had been trained to believe he was completely worthless. With that kind of a feeling, you can realize how difficult it would be to begin to like yourself.

Very few people believe the statement at first, and if you do so the first few days, be wary because your subconscious mind has a way of fooling you. A student came to me and said he had no trouble with this exercise because he had never had any doubts of liking himself. In fact, he said, he would not do it because he liked himself to such a degree it would be a waste of time. I tried to persuade him to do it anyway, but he refused. He did not make any special progress in that class. Surprisingly, he enrolled in the next class. In confidence he admitted to me that he must have done something wrong because of his lack of progress. Although he still did not feel he needed to do the mirror technique, he did it anyway. By the conclusion of the class he had uncovered several very surprising things that had been buried deep in his subconscious mind. He discovered that although on the surface he'd thought he really liked himself, it had only been a cover-up for the deep underlying feelings of rage and hostility he'd had toward his mother that he had never been able to express.

When a child has these feelings, they must be deeply hidden because children are taught that it is not "nice" to hate their mother or father. It is at this point that guilt feelings begin, and the child must then begin to suppress and cover up these deep feelings of hatred in order to be able to survive and accept himself at all. It was not a pleasant discovery for this student, but in order to dissolve these feelings permanently, it is first necessary to acknowledge they are there. Then you can forgive yourself, accept yourself as you are, and go on from there. After he did that, he made tremendous progress. These guilt feelings had been the underlying reason for his failure pattern throughout his life.

It will be wise to say to yourself many times during the day, "I like myself unconditionally," even though you do not have to look in the mirror each time. Many times when you are caught in the middle of a negative experience, it will save your day for you.

For example, if your boss has had a fight with his wife and he takes it out on you, it is not necessary to allow this to spoil your day. At that moment say silently to yourself, "I like myself unconditionally." You will be surprised at how cool and calm you will stay inside. You will be totally unaffected by the negative actions of your boss. If your spouse has a bad day and begins to attack you mentally, again use this simple technique and you will have no reaction, which will enable you to be complete master of the situation. It is always the person that does not react who has control of situations of this type.

There is one very important condition of this mirror technique. You must do this exercise for at least *twenty-one consecutive* days. If you miss even one day, you must begin your twenty-one days all over again. The reason for this period of time is that it takes a minimum of twenty-one days to form a habit, even the simplest of habits. That is what you are doing, forming a habit of liking yourself unconditionally. It would be wise to keep track of your twenty-one days on the calendar, marking off each day you do your mirror exercise. One caution: if you have had a very negative childhood, it may take much longer than twenty-one days to get a positive reaction internally. No matter how long it takes, just keep at it because eventually it will become a habit with you.

Many students ask how they will be able to tell when it finally becomes established in their subconscious mind. There will be no doubt in your mind when you like yourself unconditionally. You will have a warm, almost glowing feeling within yourself. You will be at peace with yourself. You will have no doubt at all. One test is that if you do have any doubts, you have not yet accomplished your objective of liking yourself unconditionally.

See yourself at the perfect age

The second step of this mirror image technique is the imagery part. This step is equally as important as the first one. It consists of getting yourself in a relaxed attitude through the progressive relaxation method (chapter 10), and then seeing images or pictures of yourself when you were at the age at which you would now like to spend the rest of your life. This imagery will begin to reverse your aging tendencies.

You must see as many details as possible: what time of the year it is, what time of the day it is, etc. Visualize in detail what you are wearing and what people are with you. Even imagine what smells are in the air; for example, if it is spring perhaps you can smell the hyacinths or lilacs. What sounds can you hear? Are the birds singing? Insects chirping?

Imagine this scene to yourself in exact detail. The more details you can imagine, the faster you will etch this image in your subconscious mind. The very moment it is set in your subconscious mind, your mind will begin to bring it about in your outside environment. This process can be likened to the construction of a building. The architect first has in mind the broad outline of the building he desires. He then makes a blueprint with every detail on it. The contractors take the building materials and from the blueprint begin to build it detail by detail.

This is also the process your mind goes through to bring about your wish or desire into your outside environment. First you have a broad outline of a goal, such as turning off your age. You then begin to use various techniques—first the mirror technique, then the imagery technique, filling in as many details as you can, just as the architect does with the drawing of his blueprint. You then begin to use the construction materials, such as diet and exercise, to begin to make yourself look like the youthful image you now have etched in your subconscious mind. In a matter of time, depending upon various factors such as how deeply you believe or how often you do your exercises, the image begins to take shape in your outside environment. Your friends and family may begin to say to you, long before you notice it yourself, "What have you been doing? You look so good!"

This is the simple process by which you can begin to turn off your age. It is not complicated; in fact, it really is too simple. If it could be made more difficult, many people would undoubtedly say to themselves, "I'll work very hard and accomplish this no matter how hard it is."

When things are this simple, people have a tendency to disbelieve because of the very simplicity of the techniques. Do not be misled by this. We have proof through thousands of students, not only in our Turn Off Your Age class, but also in our weight-loss classes, our Smoker's Workshops, and our Distress Workshops of the effectiveness of these techniques. If they are followed correctly, they are the key to a successful life in any area you wish to apply them.

Let me repeat, the only secret to sucess in following these procedures is *persistence*.

CHAPTER 10

In-Depth Relaxation

You have within yourself a treasure beyond belief, a pearl of such great price that if you only realized the potential of it, you would gladly spend the rest of your life learning ways to reach it—the inner depth of yourself. This great treasure is a gift to you at birth, but it is of no use until you become aware of it and learn how to use it. This magnificent gift is within all of us, without exception, and the only key to being able to use it is to become aware of it. *Awareness* is the key; and *in-depth relaxation* is the way to use it.

Uncover the gifts within yourself

The sheer simplicity and genius of such a gift is beyond the average person to comprehend. You are able to comprehend this great idea, or you would not be reading this book. Your level of consciousness has awakened you and you are inwardly aware there is something of this nature inside of you. Or at the very least, you hope there is something more within you than appears on the outside. The very fact that you have a vague feeling or a desire to explore the potential within yourself proves that you have awakened and are now ready to go on to discover the creativity within. Now there is no turning back. You will uncover all of the great and marvelous gifts within yourself, all there ready to be used, waiting only for your awareness of them.

One of the gifts is the discovery that you do not have to grow old. You will realize that this is just a world belief that is not true. The reason we know it is not true is because of the people throughout the ages who have proved to us that years and time do not mean anything. You have within you the gift of youthful maturity, the ability to watch time pass and not be affected by it.

In return for this awakening, you have an obligation. When you come to the point at which you are totally aware and have brought this awareness into all phases of your life, you must be able to pass on this knowledge. However, this will not happen until you are thoroughly aware and have made it true in your life. Then you must be an example to the world. This is the only true way of passing on knowledge, to be an example.

How does one go about bringing this awareness into the everyday facets of living? How will you bring forth this gift within yourself into your job, into your family life, into your social life? Great ideas are of no use if you cannot use them everyday in all phases of your life.

Strangely enough, the way to tap this tremendous resource within yourself involves a very simple technique. The way is *in-depth relaxation*: to learn how to relax within yourself to such a depth that when the world around you is in a turmoil, you are completely unaffected. You will feel only deep peace and contentment.

Learn to relax

Let us begin to learn the skill of relaxation. That is what relaxation is, a skill that must be practiced just as every other skill is practiced and learned, such as swimming, golf, bowling, etc.

When learning the skill of relaxation, one must first be aware of the many tense moments during the day—moments that we are not usually aware of, because in our society tension is a way of life. This tension, unfortunately, is also the very thing that keeps us from tapping into the great resources within our being. So first we must be aware of the tension before we can get the feeling of relaxation. Isn't that a paradox, that we must first recognize tension before we can recognize relaxation? Other societies throughout the world do not have this problem to the degree we have it in Western society. We have the most stress-producing society in the world. But since we love it even with all of the problems and would not be happy anywhere else, the only alternative is to learn to cope with tension by learning to relax.

This is tension

A simple demonstration of tension is to hold both arms straight out in front of you. Close both fists very tightly. The muscular contractions you feel up to your shoulders are tension. Now, direct your attention to your jaw, clench your teeth, frown as hard as you can. Now close your eyes as tightly as you can. *This is tension*! Tense your stomach muscles as hard as you can. Tense your leg muscles down to your toes. *This is tension*!

Remember, tension is muscular contraction, and relaxation is muscular limpness. Research has proved that if you can keep your muscles from contracting, you will not get tense, but will remain relaxed, no matter what the situation may be around you. Your place of employment may be in chaos, your home may be a battleground, but as long as you remain relaxed, none of this will affect you in any way. Also, as long as you remain relaxed and do not react to turmoil, the people around you will instinctively feel that you are in control of the situation.

A word of caution here. This feeling of relaxation must be genuine. It cannot be the way many people fake it. That is, they seem to be calm on the outside, but inside they are churning. Ulcers, heart attacks, and digestive upsets are among some of the penalties of this type of behavior. No, it must be a genuine feeling of total relaxation within and this cannot be faked. You may be able to fool other people, but you cannot fool your body and eventually you will pay for this deception in the form of a physical breakdown in one form or another.

Progressive relaxation

At least once a day, twice if you can manage it, practice the following progressive relaxation technique.

1. Sit down with your eyes closed and your hands resting on your knees. Concentrate your attention first on the right hand, allowing the muscles to relax, and then on the left hand, allowing the muscles to relax. Notice the word *allowing*. This means you are not to try to force yourself to get limp. It cannot be done. You must use passive relaxation, not active relaxation. Passive relaxation means to "let" the muscles relax. The word *relax* is of Latin origin. It literally means to release, to let go. So for our use, relaxing means setting free the energy that circulates within us, the same energy that operates against us every time we become nervous or upset.

2. Now with your hands relaxed, focus your attention on your arms, allowing your arms to relax.

3. Focus your attention on the top of your head and travel down your neck, shoulders, back, waist, abdominal muscles, thighs, legs, right down to the tips of your toes. Each muscle should be allowed to relax in turn. Then become aware of the weight of your body and just let this weight become limp.

4. This act of allowing each muscle to relax in turn will reveal to you the secret of shutting out the outer world and becoming aware of your inner self—a completely new experience for many people. This creativity within you is the pearl of great price. This "you" is the hub of the great potential and talents that up to this moment have remained hidden. This is your real

self, the self you were born with, the self that has no negativity, no fears of failures, no anxieties or worries. In fact, the "you" in the center of your being is at perfect peace at all times.

New sensations

When you have practiced this exercise a few times, you will become aware of two new sensations. First, it will appear to you that it is almost impossible to move. The simple thought of raising even one hand will mean a tremendous effort. This is proof that your fatigue is real, it literally has you "nailed to the ground." Second, you will become aware of a delicious inner warmth flowing within you, a feeling of complete and total peace. This is proof that you are completely relaxed. When you have this feeling, allow it to flow through you for a few moments before you go back to the business at hand.

You will find that ten minutes of this type of relaxation will allow you to do twice, even three times, as much work as you do ordinarily. It is well worth the few moments spent.

Another very simple device to allow you to relax is the act of stretching. Animals, especially cats, seem to have been born with the instinct to stretch, thus relaxing the muscles. So when you begin to feel tense, put your hands above your head and just stretch. Stand on your toes and stretch every muscle. Then allow them to go limp. This is teaching you to become aware of the difference in the feelings of tenseness and relaxation.

These appear to be such simple techniques that you may be tempted to dismiss them lightly, thinking that they are not important. Do not be fooled or misled by their very simplicity.

Let me relate the experience of a student. She thought these exercises were too simple but decided to do them anyway because she'd paid her tuition and wanted to get the most out of the class. But she did them only half-heartedly. The next day she reported to the class a strange experience. She had been sitting watching a movie on television. The movie was a humorous one with Robert Redford, the star, chasing sheep on a motorcycle. Suddenly she became aware that her muscles were beginning to tense up. Surprised, she did not attempt to do anything except to become aware, because this was the first time she'd ever noticed herself become tense from watching an interesting movie. From that time on she was able to relax herself the moment she became aware of the first tiny signs of tension.

Tension and stress are "old-age makers." Dermatologists have found that continued tension actually shears away fat deposits under the skin of the face. This causes the face to fall into wrinkles. Dr. Thomas Szasz and Alan Robertson of the University of Chicago have found that sustained tension in the jaw and scalp muscles can cause baldness by pinching the blood vessels that feed the scalp. Men with serious taut facial expressions seem to be the most affected by premature baldness.

Another exercise

Another exercise to help you relax is to have someone read the following exercise to you while you are lying down.

With the eyes open:

1. Tense both hands and arms. . . (pause). . . Now relax all tension, release all pressure and place this area of the body into a deep state of relaxation.

2. Gently contract and tense the muscles of your forehead and around your eyes. . . (pause). . . Now relax all tension, release all pressures.

3. Now gently tense the muscles of your jaw and around your mouth. . . (pause). . . Now relax all tension, release all pressures.

4. Gently tense the muscles of your shoulders and back. . . (pause). . . Now relax all tension, release all pressure and place those areas of your body into a deep state of relaxation, going deeper and deeper every time you practice this exercise.

5. Now take a deep breath and feel your chest relax as you inhale.

6. Gently tense the stomach muscles. . . (pause). . . Relax all organs, glands, even the cells and allow them to function in a normal manner.

7. Now relax the chest and stomach internally. . . (pause). . . relax deeply.

8. Tense the hips, legs, calves, and ankles. . . (pause). . . now relax the hips, legs, calves, and ankles.

9. Tense the feet and toes. . . (pause). . . Now relax the feet and toes.

10. Now relax the entire body from the top of the head all the way down to the tips of your toes.

Imagine a wave of relaxation like the waves of the ocean sweeping over you completely from the top of your head to the tips of your toes.

Repeat the above exercise with the eyes closed.

These are a few of the techniques and exercises you can teach yourself to relax with.

Again let me remind you that relaxation is the only way to reach the subconscious level of your mind. It is the only way to contact that "inner" you. It is worth all the effort it takes to learn the simple art of relaxation. The rewards are almost beyond your imagination.

CHAPTER 11

Expanding Your Reach

Suppose you had an article on a shelf that was just a little beyond your reach. What would you do? Would you stretch yourself to your full height and try to grasp it? If your fingertips just barely touched it, you'd probably try to jump a few inches in the hope of being able to get hold of it. We do this all the time in a physical type of situation. How about trying the same effort in a mental situation? That is, trying to stretch as far as you can mentally and even jumping a few inches to expand your mental reach?

Rewards are great

The rewards are great for those who make this effort, such as recognition of the great and tremendous powers within, the creativity, the potential you have never believed you have. The recognition that you have a great gift, the gift of youthful maturity, is the key to allowing the creativity to flow from within you, allowing the youthful maturity to show on the outside.

We have hundreds of stories that could be told about almost miraculous things students have done after this recognition and awareness of the storehouse of potential witin themselves. Of course after the recognition must come the action.

One student had two children and a very unhappy marriage. Her husband was alcoholic, a wonderful person when sober, but a beast when drunk. The wife and two children were in terror all through his drinking bouts. You can well imagine the low self-esteem of the wife when she began our classes. She was only 42, but looked 62. After she had used these principles and begun to realize that she had within herself a well-spring of ever-flowing creativity, miraculous things began to happen. The family had very little money. One day, out of the resources of her inner being, came this idea: "How about gathering the seed and pods and driftwood that were so abundant, painting them gold, silver or copper, and selling them? Floral arrangements could be made of dried weeds, and candelabrums for the holidays." She did this and the floral pieces were absolutely breathtaking. She had a genius for color and balance. She took a sample to a chain store in her area and they immediately ordered twelve dozen for each store. The dried weed arrangements were called "Nature's Treasures." This was a very profitable idea because her only expense was the paint. She and her children painted them and delivered them to the stores.

As she grew more and more successful, her thinking became more and more creative. She was able to reverse her age and looked much younger than her age. Unfortunately her husband did not live long enough to see the results of her creative thinking.

How did this student bring forth ideas like this from her inner being? What procedure did she use to reverse the aging tendencies brought about by her unhappy life?

She began first by a recognition that she was much more than a physical body or even a mind. She recognized that within her was power beyond belief that she had but to learn how to use. She learned not to react to her outer circumstances by using the technique of relaxation. She learned to appreciate and recognize her own inner resources. Her self-image was raised by the mirror technique. She set goals for herself, and, most important, she expanded her reach by using her creative imagination.

She visualized herself being successful each and every day no matter how negative the day was. She sat down at the same time each day, relaxed deeply, and saw pictures of herself being successful. She saw herself not only with enough money for daily needs, but also as peaceful and self-fulfilled, youthful and confident. In other words, she would imagine in her mind all of the things she was not at the moment. She did this faithfully at least once a day and often two and three times a day. The more negative and trying her day was, the more often she retreated into the inner recesses of her mind. There, deep within herself, she changed the outer appearances and made them the way she wanted them to be.

Then things began to happen. First came the idea of using dried seeds and pods as decorations for resale to stores. Then, because of the additional income, she was able to have better food for her family. The entire situation began to improve the moment she reversed the pictures in her mind of herself and her children being abused by her husband. Instead positive happy pictures of an ideal life were substituted. The student was using this as an escape from her outer conditions, but because of the process through which the mind works, in time it also became an actuality.

You cannot set goals for others

The student was very careful to set goals and use her creative imagination only for the things she herself wanted. She did not do any imagery for her husband. This is a principle taught in our classes that you must be very aware of: you cannot set any goals or visualize anything for someone else. Each person is a free agent and you cannot take away his freedom by deciding that another way of life would be best for him, even if it is a good way of life. We learn through our problems and troubles, and sometimes if you relieve someone of a problem, you have also taken away an opportunity for a great lesson of life.

An example of this was a man whose wife was alcoholic. He had read a few books about how the mind works and how to set goals and work with his creative imagination. In this case a little knowledge was worse than no knowledge. He set goals for his wife without her knowing it and used his imagery to see her sober, his family as happy and contented. For a few weeks the situation seemed to improve. His wife drank very little. Then all hell broke loose! Suddenly his wife drank more than before and was very abusive to him and to the small children. It was at this time he joined the classes, very distraught, not knowing what to do.

It was quickly explained to him that she had an inner conflict and compulsion to live the life she had and nothing he could do would change it. He could change himself, but he could never change anyone else. He could remove himself and his children from the situation, but he could not set goals for his wife and use the power of his mind to make them come true. The moment he'd attempted to do this he had hit against her mind barrier, which in a short time subconsciously aroused an antagonistic attitude within her. Because this happened on the subconscious level of her mind, she did not understand why she suddenly became so rebellious.

The husband quickly stopped setting goals for his wife and concentrated all his efforts on changing his own inner attitudes, using the mind principles in the proper and positive way.

This story had a happy ending. When the man changed himself and no longer reacted in a negative way, the wife began to lose her rebellion and one day announced she wanted to seek help from Alcoholics Anonymous. This fine group of people helped her out of the pit of alcoholism and after about two years they had a happy family. This happened not because the man changed his wife, but because he changed himself. The change in him created a desire in her to change her attitude. *Change yourself and you change your world!* Naturally one of the best side benefits was that both this man and his wife looked and acted years younger.

Expand your mental reach

This then is how you expand your mental reach, by each day picturing the type of life you wish for yourself. Every day, at the same time, sit in your favorite chair. Try to make arrangements not to be interrupted for at least ten or fifteen minutes. Take the phone off the hook. Get comfortable: take off your shoes if they are too tight, loosen your belt, take off your eye glasses, take off your earrings. In other words, if there is anything that is keeping you from feeling relaxed and comfortable, remove it so you can become totally unaware of your body or clothing. Your feet should be flat on the floor with your hands loosely in your lap. Close your eyes and begin to consciously relax yourself. Begin at the top of your head and allow the feeling of relaxation to flow throughout your body. At first you will have to focus on each muscle and allow it to relax. Tense each muscle in turn and then let it go. You will find as you practice this will begin to be an automatic process.

Begin now by taking three deep breaths, deep to the bottom of your lungs. On the fourth breath, while exhaling, mentally repeat the word *relax* to yourself several times. To enter a deeper level of relaxation, take another deep breath and mentally repeat the word *relax* as you are exhaling. To enter an even deeper, more extended level of your mind, relax all areas of your body, beginning at your head and scalp.

As you relax down through each area of your body, you will reach a deeper and deeper level of your mind.

Take another deep breath and mentally repeat the word *within* as you exhale. The cue words are *relax within*. These words are used for a special reason. The word *relax* is one we are all familiar with, and our muscles automatically begin to let go when we say the word *relax*. The word *within* is for the purpose of making you realize that the work is within yourself, not in your outside environment or from other people. No, this is strictly a "do-it-yourself" project. There is no one in this world that can reach inside your mind and turn off the switch that says, "I am getting older each day." You must do that yourself!

A key phrase

Begin by saying the words *relax within* several times to yourself. You will notice after a few days that you will automatically get a feeling of deep inner relaxation as you say these words.

At this point, in order to help you relax more easily, begin to use your creative imaginatinn. Picture to yourself three large wheels of graduated sizes. The first one is the largest, the next one a little smaller, and the third wheel the smallest one. Picture these wheels revolving very fast at first. As you begin to relax from the top of your head to the tips of your toes, the wheels begin to revolve more and more slowly. When they have completely stopped you will be at a deep level of relaxation. Then picture your goal of youthful maturity.

Now, with your creative imagination relax your

scalp and the top of your head. Imagine relaxing your forehead and facial muscles. Allow your teeth to separate slightly. Allow this sensation of relaxation to flow slowly downward throughout the body, all the way down to the toes.

Now imagine relaxing your neck and shoulders, your arms and hands. Imagine this relaxation slowly flowing downward. The "wheels" are beginning to slow down and are now turning more and more slowly. To help you keep your thoughts from intruding you may say to yourself a neutral word, such as the word *one*. This helps to keep thoughts such as "Did I turn off the gas?" or "What will I do about the knock in the car engine?" from intruding in your mind as you are trying to relax. You should never attempt to keep thoughts from entering your mind, but you should be the one who decides what kind of thoughts should be there. In other words, you must learn to discipline your mind. This is one of the most important aspects of this relaxation exercise.

Now imagine relaxing your back muscles, your chest muscles, and your abdominal muscles; imagine this relaxation flowing downward, all the way down to your toes. Imagine now relaxing down through your hips and legs, through the calves and feet, all the way down to your toes. It is a pleasant feeling to be so deeply relaxed. You are now in a deeper, more extended level of your subconscious mind. The wheels are turning very, very slowly now.

To enter a deeper, still more extended level, imagine yourself in a serene relaxing setting, your ideal place of relaxation, wherever that may be. It may be on a beautiful pure white sandy beach, high up in the mountains among the tall pines, beside a peaceful river, or even in your own home. Whatever your ideal place of relaxation may be, imagine yourself there now. Spend at least three or four minutes there and allow yourself to relax even more completely. Take a deep breath and enter an even deeper level, with the wheels revolving ever so slowly. Now you notice the wheels have stopped completely and you are in a very deep, deep expanded level of consciousness.

As you are in this dreamlike state, imagine yourself at the age at which you would like to spend the rest of your life. Pull out of your memory a period of your life when you were very happy and contented. Relive that period of your life, adding to it anything you might like to have changed. See this scene in every detail. See yourself laughing, talking, feeling the marvelous sensations of exuberance beginning to flow within you. You realize that you have within you the capacity to turn off your age. But more than that, you now realize that in a short period of time you can even reverse your age characteristics. You realize what a great and marvelous instrument you have in the power of your mind.

You realize there is nothing you cannot do if you follow the principles you have learned. You have reached within you that deep, deep center of your being that is never disturbed by outer conditions, that can only be reached by deep relaxation.

You are in control

The feeling of joy within you almost overwhelms you as you now know for a certainty that you are in control of your body. You now know that through the discipline of your mind you can have the best of both worlds: the energy, vitality, and exuberance of youth plus the wisdom, calmness, and maturity of experience. You can have for the rest of your life *youthful maturity*.

From now on, that feeling of joy and vitality will be yours. You will be dynamically alive. Your image of your old body is fading and the image of your new youthful body is getting stronger and stronger. Your present physical body is merging into the new youthful mold. You are now, at this very moment, moving toward the realization of this body and mind of youthful maturity. Henceforth you will be doing whatever is needed to achieve this as quickly as possible. You will have a better environment, better nutrition, an exercise program. Anything that needs to be done to more quickly help you achieve your goal of youthful maturity will now begin and nothing will stand in your way.

This ideal model will exist in your subconscious mind at all times, existing there as a magnetic attracting force, a vital force that will draw and compel you to do whatever is necessary until you have achieved your goal of youthful maturity.

Now, using your creative imagination, visualize yourself doing all the things necessary for obtaining this goal as quickly as possible. See yourself doing exercise and enjoying it. See yourself eating wholesome nutritious foods and taking supplements. See yourself doing the things you enjoy doing, things that keep your mind and body active. See yourself surrounded by friends and family who love you. Also see yourself enjoying times when you are alone. See yourself in an activity of helping others because you must feel needed. Most of all, feel that deep feeling of contentment, that deep inner feeling of self-fulfillment, that is the only true peace.

Now say the master affirmation, *"I like myself unconditionally"* three times.

Slowly stretch your arms over your head, flex your muscles and you will be out of the subconscious level of your mind. Do this exercise at least once a day and twice if possible.

Each time you practice this mental exercise, you are making a pattern in your brain cells. You are making a blueprint in your mind of your goal of youthful maturity. The more you practice this, the sooner it will come about. Your subconscious mind has the power to bring about in your outer environment anything you can picture to yourself. The moment it is firmly entrenched in your subconscious mind, your goal will be completed and you will have what you most desire, youthful maturity.

So begin this very moment by expanding your mental reach, remembering that each time you practice, your reach is getting longer and longer and soon you will grasp this wonderful goal of remaining forever youthful.

CHAPTER 12

Time is Your Tool

Until this moment you may have thought that time is your enemy; that with each passing day, month, and year you are getting older and older. I hope that you are now beginning to realize that you and you alone have complete and absolute control of your mind, and through discipline of your mind, control of your body.

Time is your tool because with each passing day you are acquiring new knowledge and inner awareness and releasing your creativity. This in turn is giving you inner strength, inner peace, and inner confidence. You are beginning to realize that within you is the potential for limitless possibilities. You are beginning to grasp the exciting reality that you, by using the simple tools presented in this book, can bring this great inner power into your outside world.

Share your awareness

There is a condition that must be met when this newfound awareness is an actual part of you. Notice that I say it must be an "actual part of you." When this happens and the teaching is the very fiber of your being, you then share it with others. You must always give away anything you have discovered within yourself. If you do not do this, you will not be able to retain your new knowledge. Many teachers have found that when they teach they always learn more than the students. Inner knowledge has a way of compounding within when you impart it without. However, a very strict warning: you must be absolutely sure that it is actually your inner realization. You cannot proselytize, but you must demonstrate what you believe. You must be a living example. That is the only true way of teaching. If you would tell others to turn off their age, you must be a true example of vitality, energy, and enthusiasm.

Time is of whatever value you put on it. This is what is meant by the phrase, "Time is your tool." If you put a positive value on it and use time wisely in getting an inner realization of your great potential, an awareness of the fact that you have control of your life, then time will be working for you. If, on the other hand, you use time to bemoan the fact that things are not the way you'd like them to be, that you are getting older with each passing day, then time is working against you. Realize that you and you alone make this decision. You make the choice whether time will work for you or against you.

A living example of this is Dr. Keith E. Good, who

had already earned several degrees when at age 72 he received a bachelor's degree in psychology. This in itself is most unusual, but even more so is that he received a straight "A" average for 76 semester hours of study. His plans now are to seek a master's degree in psychology at a California institution, and retirement is not his goal. Dr. Good is living proof of the "total" living concept that has been presented in each chapter. He is an avid reader and regular participant in weekly exercise and swimming exercises for senior citizens. "Among my peers, those who follow some type of program are alert. Those who retire physically and mentally are deteriorating," Dr. Good said, adding, "The mind is like concrete. If it is not stirred up occasionally, it will set-up." Dr. Good is making time his tool to achieve all of the things he has been interested in in his entire life, while still carrying on an active medical practice.

William R. McKie, an incredibly spry 108, also has goals ahead of him yet. When he was asked by a reporter, "What keeps you ticking?" he said, "I still got a lot of fishing to do." Mr McKie is also making time his tool instead of allowing it to work against him.

Strive for a goal

Discipline yourself to think of time as very valuable to you instead of as working against you. In order to make time valuable, you must set goals. You must have something ahead of you, just as Dr. Good does. Although he received one college degree, he is now setting a goal for another one, and we have no doubt when he achieves that one, still another goal will be ahead of him. That is the secret, to have goals and achievements to work for. The striving for a goal is the ultimate of pleasures. When you finally obtain your goal, it is a secondary thing. The striving is the real pleasure. So the moment you achieve one goal, immediately set another one.

Dr. Good did some very interesting research while studying for his degree. He found that there are only two groups in the world that treat their elders without respect: the United States and some Eskimos. Some Eskimos take care of their older population by putting them on ice floes when they are no longer able to handle their share of the work. A polar bear usually discovers them and this achieves two goals, that of taking care of the elder and also of having the bear stay around the habitation so the rest of the tribe can kill the bear to supply them with their meat for the winter. Dr. Good compares this with our nation's solution of putting the elders in nursing homes. He said this is the equivalent of the Eskimos' ice floe.

If we do not want to be put on an "ice floe" we must begin now a "do-it-yourself" program to turn off our age. No one will do it for us. Do not believe that you are too young to be concerned about aging. Even people in their early 20s should begin to reverse their thinking about aging at this very moment.

An excellent example of this type of thinking was brought to the attention of the class by a student in a "Turn Off Your Age" seminar. She was 24 years young at that time, a beautiful dark-haired woman. She took it very seriously when we advised the class that *now* is the time to begin to reverse the "aging thinking." She determined to "freeze" her age at age 24. She practiced faithfully the exercises taught in the class and now, twelve years later at the so-called age of 36, she still looks 24. She has three sons from ages 10 to 16 whom she is raising alone. Whenever anyone sees her, they are amazed that at her "young" age she would have a son 16. (Everyone guesses her to be in her early 20s.) Another student in a later class also took the class very seriously and faithfully practiced all that she had learned. She was 35 at that time, and now ten years later people are always guessing her to be around 28 or 29. These are beautiful examples of what can be done to not only turn off your age but also to reverse it.

Of course youthful appearance is very enjoyable, but much more important is the attitude of feeling youthful, energetic, and enthusiastic about life. That is much more important than looks. Not all the students looked as youthful as the two examples, but all the students had a very marvelous outlook toward going forward instead of looking backward.

Let go of the past

One of the first things students learn is to let go of the past completely. True, it may be referred to once in a while as an experience, but only to allow it to influence or affect the present as a "learning tool." In other words, we learn from all experiences in the past, but we never allow the past to negate our present. This means that no matter how distressing, disgraceful, or difficult the past may have been to you, you must realize that it is gone. Anyone who permits the past to influence them except as a learning tool is foolish. The past is gone, it is dead. Do not torture yourself with things that happened in the past, only learn from them. Remember never to assume guilt!

Both of the students who were mentioned as examples had very difficult past lives. The first lovely lady went through a difficult divorce, but she successfully raised her boys to be models of what ideal young men should be. The second beautiful lady also had a difficult past from which she learned. The family many times had little or nothing to eat. She also went through a difficult divorce, and even had to go on welfare for a time to have enough for her children to eat. She took this opportunity to learn from her mistakes. She went back to school and is now a registered nurse, has remarried a wonderful man, and her children are now emotionally very stable.

As you can see, most of my students do not have an easy life, but the difference between these people and the average person is that they do not sit around feeling sorry for themselves. They take action and learn from their past experiences to make a positive future for themselves. There is no situation in your life that cannot be a stepping stone to a better, happier future for you. If you have terrible problems at this moment, begin to think of them as the very things that will guide you to a marvelous future.

The first thing students are told in the classes is this: "If you have problems, bad problems, problems that make you hurt inside, rejoice, because these terrible feelings of inner pain inside you will act as a lever to make you try harder than anyone else. You will get much more out of these classes because you hurt more and you will try harder. The saddest of all people are those who float on a sea of complacency. Nothing very bad ever happens to them so they make no effort to do anything. Your problems are the very things that will make for you a glorious future if you work toward solving them in a positive way."

There are some people in their 70s and 80s, or even in their early 60s, who let the length of their years on earth spoil their todays by dwelling on how many years of the past there have been and counting how few there are left in the future. There would be more happy years in the future if they would live in the present.

Live in the present

Now is the only time there is, the only span of time your subconscious recognizes. Your subconscious mind does not recognize the past because it is gone and does not see the future because it is not here. If you are consciously bemoaning the bad experiences of the past and yearning for a future that will bring better things, stop at this very moment! Learn to live not only in "day-tight" compartments, but even in "hour-tight" compartments. Do not dwell on the past, do not yearn for the future, but do enjoy this day, this hour, this moment! There are so many things to be enjoyed: beautiful sunrises in the mornings, a glistening snowy day with the first rays of the sun painting the snow in hues of pink, orange, and violet. Listen when the first yearnings of spring begin with the songbirds singing their happiness. Then enjoy the lovely summer nights with the temperature exactly like your own so you feel as if you are floating in a sea of air and you are one with all nature.

Learn to be aware of beauties around you. Learn not to see the negative, the ugly, the sad, the depressing things. Instead teach yourself to see the beautiful, the lovely, the positive. This is a strict mind discipline you must practice because we have all been taught to see the negative. Now, at this very moment, begin to train yourself to be aware of the beauties of life.

Do not misunderstand and think you are not to plan or set goals for the future. You are to set goals for yourself, but do not be so rigid that your plans and goals cannot be changed. The only certainties about life are that there will be change and lots of it. This world is in a constant change, never quite stable. We must learn to accept the instability as normal, because it is. There is no such thing as stability in this world.

Our concern, then, is with the *now*. The only thing we have to do with tomorrow is to know that things willl come up that have to be done and we will do them then, and not worry about them today.

This is the way to make time your tool. Forget yesterday and all of the problems you had and even all of the good times. Yesterday is of no use to you except as a learning tool. Tomorrow will never come because it is always in the future. Set your positive goals for tomorrow, but do the actions today, right now, at this very moment.

Time in this way can be your tool, instead of time making you its tool.

CHAPTER 13

Keeping Curiosity Alive

There is much more to turning off your age than exercise, diet, and an optimistic outlook. As one doctor said, "All of these things are mechanical, but what of the healing powers of the mind?" The current explosion of interest in the mind has demonstrated unsuspected powers of the mind.

The mind is the starting place for turning off your age. You must first have a conscious desire to want to remain "youthfully mature" before anything else can happen. This you must already have, or you would not be reading this book.

We will begin from the premise that you have a strong desire to remain youthfully mature for the balance of your life. While reading this book, you have learned of the various experiments regarding the aging process and that there are no specific "diseases of aging." In other words, people do not necessarily die of old age, but of other diseases related to improper nutrition, insufficient exercise, no interest in life, not feeling important, and last, but most important, not having any more curiosity about anything in life.

Many interesting things

It is important to keep curiosity alive, to be interested in various facets of living. The world is so full of interesting things. There are things from the past, such as ancient history of various cultures, or the excavation of ancient cities. There are things of the present, current events that you can see on television, read about in the newspaper, or hear about on the radio. There are plans for the future, such as experiments to see if computers can be programmed to think for themselves, or plans to send space vehicles to other planets to bring soil, rocks, and other materials back to earth. There are many areas to delve into if you but keep your curiosity alive.

The dictionary defines curiosity as "an eager desire to know." An eager desire to know suggests an aliveness, a forwardness, positive vibrations throughout your body. So one of the very important steps in the process of turning off your age is to keep your curiosity alive about everything around you.

Begin at this moment, no matter how many years you've spent here on earth, to make a firm decision. Decide what you want to be curious about. It should be something you have always wondered about, but up to this moment have not done anything to investigate. The time is now, right now, to do something. Perhaps you have always been curious about your own ancestors. You can begin now to write to various places to get information. An excellent place to begin is the Genealogy Society of the Mormon Church in Salt Lake City, Utah. They have most extensive volumes of history of families over the entire world.

Perhaps you have always been curious about insects, TV game shows, or how something is made. It matters not how small or insignificant you believe it is. The important thing is that you have a desire to know more about it. Then set about in various ways to get more information. Scratch beneath the surface, look underneath to see what makes the whole thing tick. See what the undergirdings are in whatever area you are interested in. The easiest place to begin is your local public library. From there you will be able to get the information that will lead to other sources of information.

Never, never, never say to others, or even to yourself, "I can't do that, I'm too old." Those words spoken, or even thought, are like drinking a glass of pure poison. With words like that, you have sealed your own fate, and no one can help you except yourself. If, in the past, you have said similar words, right now turn them around and say to yourself and to others, "I may have mistakenly thought I was too old, but now I realize that I am ever renewing, ever looking forward to life and living. I have curiosity about many things and am taking action to find out more about them."

Say this to yourself the moment you open your eyes in the morning and the last thing at night just as you are dozing off to sleep. When you begin to dream about these words, and realize you are saying them throughout the night, then you have reversed the aging process that you yourself began with those negative words, "I'm too old."

Mental jogging

Exercising your mind, which is a sort of "mental jogging," is just as important for turning off your age as exercising your body. Curiosity is the trigger that begins the exercising of your mind. Your mind reacts exactly as your body does. If you exercise a muscle faithfully, it responds and gets stronger and stronger. At first the muscle will be weak and sore, but persistence soon pays off and the muscle is at peak form. Your mind reacts exactly the same way. If you don't exercise it, it begins to lose its abilities and you become as weak in that area as if it were an unused muscle.

You begin to have all kinds of negative emotional feelings, such as depression, anxieties, worries, self-pity, lonesomeness, etc. All of these symptoms are the signs of an unexercised mind, a mind that is lying dormant in spite of all the tremendous powers, the creativity, the potential that everyone is born with. Yes, you have been born with all of these things, but if you do nothing with them, the reaction is exactly like an unused muscle. It atrophies and is of no further use to you.

Here are ten tips to help you begin your mind jogging.

1. Subscribe to a daily newspaper and read it. If you watch TV news, realize that the mind wanders when

watching television, but when reading you must concentrate more.

2. If you watch a lot of television, begin to read books instead. Watching television is a passive activity, but books stimulate thought. Be careful not to read trash. You might read books by Hemingway, O. Henry, or Shakespeare, or books on things you are curious about.

3. If you must watch TV, skip the game shows and soap operas and watch news broadcasts, documentaries, panel discussions—shows that will set your brain to working.

4. Check to see if your church, club, or other organization has a discussion group and join it. If you can't find one, start one. There are always one or two other people who wish to begin a new journey with their life. Discuss current events so you'll know what is going on in the world.

5. Do volunteer work. Just being around people stimulates mental activity.

6. Continue your education. There are many colleges now that offer classes to the "third age" people. Check out some of the adult education classes in your community.

7. Take up a hobby and learn all you can about it. If you like gardening, for example, find out all about soil conditions, hybrids, insects that are helpful, organic conditions, etc. There is a lot more to gardening than dropping tiny seeds into holes in the ground. There is a great deal more to anything than meets the eye.

8. Make special trips to museums and art galleries in your area. When you do, don't just look at exhibits,

read the explanatory notes under them. Take notes yourself and if you see something interesting, do research on it in your library.

9. Instead of telephoning your friends, write letters instead. It is a mental exercise to write a letter. Chatting on the phone is often a waste of time.

10. For other mental stimulation when you are alone, play solitaire or solve crossword puzzles. Put together a jigsaw puzzle.

All of these things are forms of exercise for your mind and if you try even one of them, you will see for yourself in a very short time that you will be thinking much more positive thoughts and you will begin to feel alive.

All of the scientific research done in the last few years points to the fact that our bodies and minds are made to last much longer than they do. Because we are not doing the right things, we mistakenly believe we are getting old, whereas in reality it is just misuse or nonuse of either body or mind.

Get out of your rut

Inertia is the biggest stopgap to achieving "aliveness," vitality, and energy. Get out of your rut this moment; do something entirely different from your usual routine. If you always sleep late, get up at sunrise and watch the sun come up, listen to the early morning birds, feel the cool morning breeze, and listen to the quiet of the dawn. There is a holy hush at that time of the day that is not duplicated at any other time. If you always get up early, then sleep late and see how it feels. Try it, you may like it.

If you are always alone, be with other people even if it is only walking in a crowded department store. If you are always with people, make some time to be alone. If you have never been to a ballet or a concert, go and experience them. Or go to a rock concert, which is an entirely different sensation and worth experiencing at least once.

Help someone else

But most important, you must begin to feed your soul, to have an activity that is of great satisfaction to you. Such satisfaction is usually in service to one or more human beings, by helping, if only in a small way, someone who desperately needs the assistance of someone else. This requirement can be satisfied by volunteering in any one of the numerous organizations that are always in need of help.

One of the most impressive organizations I have heard of is composed of older people who are substitute grandparents for young children who have no one at home when they return from school. Their parents are working and they must come home to an empty house. The substitute grandparents either go to the house to be there when the children come home, or if they live close by, have the children come to their home. Some of the grandmothers bake cookies for their young charges or have other small surprises. The grandfathers fill the need with repairing bicycles or telling stories. The older people are needed and the children are happy to have a warm caring person there. There is nothing more lonely than for a small child to come home to an empty house. A very important need is met for both the grandparents and the children. One of the requirements for turning off your age is that you must feel needed—there must be a reason for living! Remember, you are a total person and all of the requirements must be met on all levels of living.

Remember that the law of the universe is action and change. You cannot sit on the fence and do nothing; you must have movement and change. If you do not go forward, you will retrogress and go backward. But always there is movement of some kind. If you do not take active charge of your life, you will still be moving but not in the direction you may wish to go.

So right now, at this very moment, set into motion the law of turning off your age by some kind of action, some kind of movement. Any kind will do as long as it is physical action or mental exercise. The idea is to do something completely different and opposite from your usual routine to get yourself out of your inertia. The most important thing is to do it *now*. Do not wait until tomorrow because there is no tomorrow, there is only *now*.

CHAPTER 14

It's Up To You and You Alone

As you now realize, turning off your age is strictly a do-it-yourself project. There is no one who can reach into your mind and turn off the switch that keeps saying, "I'm getting old." You must do that yourself, but as you can now see from the examples and instructions, it is surprisingly simple. You have only to use the tools that are already within yourself and put there at birth by your Creator.

All of scientific research only confirms the idea that you have been endowed with special creative processes controlled only by yourself. The key is within you. The key is realization and awareness that you have within you all the power, potential, and creativity to do this job. We have proved again and again in our classes with thousands of students that it *works!*

Your age is just a number

One very important thing to remember is that your age is just a number. It has nothing to do with how young you are. Numbers don't count, it's how you feel and what you do. That's how young you are.

Time of itself has no power to age us. It is the belief in the effects of time that ages us. This is the first link that must be broken in the chain of aging. A really serious determined effort is required to accomplish this. All through our lives we have had to unlearn many things in order to advance and learn more. A baby first learns to crawl and then has to "unlearn" how to crawl before he begins to walk. This is a natural process and requires no effort on the baby's part. We too need to unlearn a belief that we were conditioned with as children. It was a good belief up to a certain time because it helped us to mature. But like the baby's crawl, after a certain period, it is no longer a good belief and must be changed.

Now we need to recondition our minds to discard the belief that time causes aging. Time is immensely useful in enabling us to regulate our life. But should we let it control our life to the degree that we do? Should we allow this hypothetical measurement to determine the length of our life as we do now? Just because the earth swirls around the sun in approximately 365 days, are we to believe that we are therefore a year older? If we have been traveling on the earth for sixty or seventy of these trips around the sun, should we expect to die because of that? Should we say that we are "a year older," or should we just say that we have enjoyed another swing around the sun?

Our emotional reaction to this thing called "time"

has been learned from the day we were born. Our emotions can be forces for good or bad, so our emotional learned reaction to the passage of time is a definite force in our life. This emotion, housed in the mind, has a very powerful effect on the body.

Feelings about age

Let's try an experiment right now to see if we can prove this to ourselves. Sit quietly for a few moments with your eyes closed. Do not allow any noises to distract you. Now, using your creative imagination, get a "feeling" about old age in the way you were taught.

Think of your current age. Now, using your imagination, think of yourself as you were ten to twenty years ago. Remember a specific happening and recall all of the details: the time of year, what you were doing, what you were wearing, what people were there, etc. Notice the feeling of emotion when you think of yourself ten to twenty years younger. Do you have a more energetic feeling about yourself, almost a joyous feeling?

Now think of yourself as being ten or twenty years older. Do you get a sinking feeling, a depressing negative reaction? I think I can safely say that almost everyone has learned to think of getting older in negative terms.

These feelings were learned responses and not necessarily the truth of the situation at all. Perhaps in ten years you will be much happier than you are at this moment.

Now, again think of yourself ten years later, but

this time visualize yourself as just taking ten swings around the sun in a state of joy, feeling very vital, energetic, and happy. Is there a definite difference in your emotional reaction to the two ways of looking at your progress? That is the positive way of thinking of time progressing, of just thinking of yourself taking swings around the sun.

So now realize that aging begins in your mind. The aging control center in the brain appears to be the thalamus, hypothalamus and pituitary: the neuro-endocrines. If you believe you will get old at a certain period in your life, or you lose interest in life, an imbalance in the serotonin and norepinephrine (the neurotransmitters in the brain) soon appears. This imbalance is believed to be the trigger of the physical appearance of old age. The imbalance also activates or speeds up the overall rate of aging.

Don't throw the switch

The very moment you have the "old age" belief, you yourself throw the switch in the very heart of the brain that will throw you into an hormonally induced aging decline. You alone have the control at your fingertips to either stop, reverse, or allow the aging process in your body.

How can you not only "freeze your age" but also reverse the aging tendencies? Dr. Hans Kugler, an anti-ageing researchers and author of *Slowing Down the Ageing Process*, confirms research findings of Dr. Benjamin Frank, and also the research being done at Duke University. All agree that much can be accomplished through first of all having the correct, positive attitude toward aging. The next essential requirements for "turning off your age" are exercise and good nutrition. You must have positive goals in your life, a curiosity for life, a zest for living. Always realize you are here on earth for a purpose; you have something that must be accomplished. Find out what it is.

You can begin to find out this "reason for being" by searching out first of all what interests you more than anything else. Pinpoint whatever that interest is, no matter how small or trivial you may think it is. Remember great oaks come from small acorns. If through honest introspection you decide that nothing interests you, you will have to jolt yourself into reactivating an interest you may have once had. If you do not have any interests, you have already allowed the control center in your brain to begin shutting down your body machinery. But remember, this can be reversed almost at once by cultivating an interest in something, anything, no matter how small or insignificant. It can be just a small plant you are helping to grow and nurture, or birds you are helping keep alive during a hard winter. It matters not what it is, it just matters that you do it.

One student of over 70 revived an interest in his home. He'd been active years before in fixing things here and there. Suddenly he allowed the control center of the mind to begin the "aging" process. He lost interest in everything. After attending the class, he realized that he himself had allowed this, so he once more began to work and repair his home. He became interested in installing a solar system for hot water. He went to the library, took classes to learn how to do it, and talked to many experts in the field. It took him over a year to install his solar system, but in that time he reversed his aging tendencies by ten years. When he renewed his interest in his home he automatically got more exercise by walking and building the solar system. He gave heed to the nutrition part of the "de-aging" process and began to eat much better. But most important of all, he realized that he alone had the power to turn off the "aging" switch in his mind and he did it! He became such an expert that he is now a consultant in helping other people to install "do-it-yourself" solar systems in their homes—a new career at the so-called age of 83.

Does this remind you of another youthful chap who began a career at age 65 and is still going strong almost twenty years later? You've seen this energetic man on television. Yes, Colonel Sanders began his career of selling fried chicken when he got his first Social Security check and vowed he would not sit in a rocking chair for the rest of his life and attempt to exist on that meager check. He realized he was created for something much greater than that and he did it. This is a marvelous example of an interest that may seem rather small and insignificant to many people. A recipe for fried chicken does not sound like the beginning of a worldwide career, but it was.

So no matter how tiny you may think your interest is at first, do not discount it; it may be the beginning of a worldwide career for you also! But you must remember that only you can make the vow to make the "third age" of your life one of the most interesting and rewarding.

CHAPTER 15

Mind Resistance

There is a strange phenomenon that will happen when you begin your program to turn off your age. It is something you must be aware of. If you are not aware of it, it will defeat you before you even begin.

Recent research has uncovered something that has been named "mind resistance." It works in this fashion.

Your mind at first will resist your efforts to begin your program. You may find all sorts of "garbage" beginning to float up to your conscious awareness from your subconscious mind—things such as "you're too old to begin a program of this kind at your age," or "it's absolutely ridiculous to think of doing something of this magnitude," or "Forget it Charlie, your relatives all aged at an early age," or "you don't have the stick-to-it-iveness to do this, don't bother to even begin."

What do you have to lose?

All negative thoughts of this nature are *gar-bage*. You were conditioned and programmed to believe this type of nonsense. Recognize this at once! Push your way through such nonsense; do not let it stop you. After all, what do you have to lose by beginning this program to turn off your age? Anything? If you never get anywhere with it, you will be no worse off than you are at this moment, and if you do get somewhere, you can only gain and be a winner. In other words, this Turn Off Your Age program is a winner's game. You cannot lose, so begin now at this very moment to turn off the switch in your mind that keeps telling you erroneously that day by day you are getting older.

Not too many years ago a fad called "sleep teaching" was very popular. It consisted of buying a program with a series of tapes of whatever you wished to learn during the time you were asleep. You just put the speaker under your pillow, and, presto, in the morning you could converse fluently in German or Russian or whatever you wanted to learn!

Unfortunately after a week or ten days, many people got discouraged and decided it would not work and so discontinued it. In those days it was not known that the mind has a barrier that has to be considered before a program of this nature, and with suitable subject matter, can be successful. There are only about twenty to thirty minutes when you fall asleep and about the same amount of time when you awaken in which you can learn. It is in only that short period that learning of this type can take place.

It takes from three to four weeks to break through the mind barrier. The mind barrier or resistance consists of your subconscious mind telling you that "it won't work, so why even bother to try," or "you were silly to spend good money on such a stupid thing," and on and on with all kinds of negative statements.

Simply stated, that is all the mind barrier or resistance is: all of the negative statements, attitudes, and concepts you were taught as a child. They are so strong and so entwined that it seems as if you have an impregnable barrier in your mind. It is at this point that you give up in a few days and do not try again.

Persist and succeed

If, however, you are aware that this very thing will happen, you will not give up, but will try much harder. If you persist, in just a few days you will break through your mind resistance and it will not bother you again. In the very process of becoming aware of this barrier, you will succeed in penetrating it perhaps for the first time in your life. This is how you have made yourself a prisoner of your own mind.

A student told this story in a class a short time ago. She knew she had a very strong desire to turn off her age and did not really pay too much attention to warnings about the mind resistance. After doing her mental exercises for two weeks, one day she woke up with the most depressed feelings and the thoughts that came to her were, "It won't work, why even bother to keep it up?" Another thought that kept popping in her mind was that she was not worthy to look good, so why did she go to all this trouble? Immediately she recognized that she had hit very hard against the mind barrier and she then redoubled her efforts and in two days broke through the resistance and had no problems with it after that.

There have been other students who have had repeated problems hitting against the mind resistance. Each time they break through, they encounter it again in a week. These students have had extremely negative conditioning in their childhood, with backgrounds of total rejection, brutality, alcoholism, etc. It becomes very difficult for them to have any feelings of worthiness at all. But even·they, in a matter of months, eventually break through this barrier. Fortunately, this type of childhood conditioning is the exception rather than the rule.

Just keep in mind that each time you begin to have feelings of doubt, inertia, or depression, these are false feelings, attitudes, and concepts still trying to control you from your early childhood days. Your old emotional patterns will keep coming back time after time unless you consciously become involved in a program of self-improvement of some type.

If you do nothing else, begin with the mirror technique each day for twenty-one days and at the end of that time you will have the necessary confidence to begin the rest of the de-aging process. This technique alone will erase many of the feelings of "it won't work" or "I am not worthy to look good," etc. The mere fact of being aware of this mind barrier resistance will erase three-fourths of the problems you would have had otherwise. Awareness of anything is always three-fourths of the battle won.

CHAPTER 16

Let's Tie It All Together

Now let's tie all of the information together that has been presented in this book. You will then have a sequence of procedures that you can do each day in order to begin at once your action program of turning off your age.

I. Mental exercises

A. MIRROR TECHNIQUE

1. Each morning as soon as you wake up, go to your mirror and look directly into your eyes (ignore the image of your face). Say out loud with much enthusiasm, **"I like myself unconditionally."** Say it to yourself as many times during the day as you can remember. (You only have to say it out loud while looking in the mirror twice during the day.) You must

do this for a minimum of twenty-one days in order to form a habit of liking yourself. In order to remind yourself to say it often, write it on several 3 x 5 cards and tape them wherever you will be looking, such as the dashboard of your car, your desk, the front of the refrigerator, your bathroom mirror, etc.

B. EXPANDING YOUR CREATIVE IMAGINATION

1. At least once during the day, retire to a quiet place and expand your creative imagination by relaxing thoroughly with the relaxation exercise in chapter 10. Use your imagination to visualize a goal you would like, yourself at the age you would like to return to, or a very happy time in your life. Any one of these images will generate a very happy feeling for you for the rest of the day.

The best time to do this exercise is during the low-energy part of your day. This is usually during the afternoon if you are a morning person, or, mid-morning if you are an evening person. Another excellent time is right after you come home from a long hard day in your place of employment. However, any time you have about ten to fifteen minutes of quiet in the day will do very nicely.

You will also find that you are tapping into the energy level of your mind and you will awaken from this exercise with a feeling of relaxed and controlled energy. Many students, after they have practiced this for a few weeks, have reported they do not have to sleep as many hours during the night as before and they have much more energy during the day. The reason for increased energy is that the negative, depressing, worried thoughts are being erased, releasing a great deal of energy for projects that are much more worthwhile. If you find yourself having difficulty doing this deep relaxation that is so necessary for success in this program, you will find on the last page of this book a list of cassette tapes that have proved to be very helpful for students.

II. Physical exercises

A. You have now decided on the best exercise program for yourself, so be very faithful in doing this each day, or at the very least, three times a week for fifteen minutes at a time. (It can be longer if you wish, but it should not be less.) If you are jogging, you will need to jog at least three days during the week. The stretching exercises should be done each day when you finish taking your bath or shower. Remember also to exercise your face, as there are many muscles there. The jump rope exercise also needs to be practiced at least three times a week for fifteen minutes after you have slowly worked up to that amount of time. Do not try to jump fifteen minutes at first. Begin with just one minute, increasing to two minutes the next week, and so on until you reach fifteen minutes.

I have found a good exercise program is to alternate exercises. Three times a week I jog if the weather is good. If it is bad weather, I jump rope inside instead. The other three days I pick whatever appeals to me the most—swimming, bicycling, tennis, or any other sport that is appealing. Stretching I do every day because it feels so good. On the seventh day I rest.

III. Nourishment that produces high energy

1. Each day eat one egg, one piece of whole grain bread with butter.

2. Drink one glass of fresh vegetable juice, juiced with a vegetable juicer.

3. Drink two glasses of skim milk (if you are watching your weight) with 1 tablespoon of acidophilus stirred into each glass.

4. Use yogurt freely. In place of sour cream in tartar sauce, it can be spooned over broiled or baked fish fillets before putting in the oven. You can also stir fresh fruit or raisins, nuts, etc. into the yogurt.

5. Four to six times a week, eat a small can of sardines, packed in water, if you are watching your calorie intake. On the other days have another type of fish. You may have calves' liver once a week and poultry once a week.

Beef will be on your menu only once a week. In other words, you are changing the percentage of protein from mostly animal meats to mostly fish. Formerly you ate 90 percent meat to 10 percent fish; now it should be 90 percent fish to 10 percent meat. You should not do this overnight, however, Change your eating habits gradually. If you have not eaten much fish during your life, just begin eating fish two or three times a week for the first month, than each week add another fish meal until at the end of six months you are eating the correct percentage of fish to meat.

6. Once a day eat one of the following: radishes, onions, mushrooms, spinach, celery, cauliflower, or asparagus.

7. Once or twice a week eat peas, lima beans, lentils, soybeans, or beets.

8. Once a day have a green salad with as many fresh vegetables as you can put in it. Use an oil and vinegar dressing or lemon and oil. Or you may make a dressing out of yogurt such as the following:

½ cucumber, peeled and cut into small chunks
1 cup yogurt
1 teaspoon white vinegar
¼ teaspoon seasoned salt
1 small clove garlic, chopped
1 tomato (medium)
½ cup minced onion

Whirl cucumber, yogurt, vinegar, salt, and garlic in blender until pureed. Peel tomato and chop fine. Add tomato and onion to yogurt mixture. Chill for several hours for best flavor. Makes 2½ cups and is only 5 calories per tablespoon.

9. Each day take a therapeutic strength multi-vitamin after any one of the meals. Use a vitamin of a good brand and good reputation.

10. Drink at least four glasses of water per day.

You may sprinkle 1 to 2 teaspoons of wheat germ, lecithin, and brewer's yeast on any salad, or you can stir any of them into a vegetable drink.

The only strict rule of this diet is never neglect to drink your two glasses of milk, one glass of vegetable juice, and four glasses of water per day. **This is a must**! The reason for this is that this way of eating may cause complications for the small percentage of people who have high blood-uric acid levels. There are people who may have a tendency toward kidney stone or gout. A word of caution, however: always check with your doctor about any change in your diet, particularly if you are already following a diet. Your doctor knows you and your needs.

IV. Spiritual Exercises

A. Each day before even getting out of bed, take just a moment to be grateful for the positive things in your life. Realize that you are not alone. There is always an influence, your Creative Source, that is with you if you will but allow yourself to become aware of it.

B. At least once a day forgive anyone who has aroused any negative feelings within you. Most of all, forgive yourself for any mistakes or blunders you might have made. We all do the best we can with the knowledge and experience we have at the moment. Do not condemn yourself; you did the best you could.

V. Action Exercises

A. Remember to keep your curiosity alive. Each day something must be done that is different from your usual routine. You may have to force yourself for the first twenty-one days, but after that it will become a habit and you will no longer have to even think about it. It will then be so automatic that you will miss it if you do not do it.

One word of caution. Do keep this program a secret for the first twenty-one days at least. There are too many negative people who will doubt you and make you doubt yourself if you tell them what you intend to do. They will immediately say that it will not work and because at this moment you are not completely sure that it will work either, you may believe them and then will not even begin the program.

It has also been found in our class work that the energy you get inside from the enthusiasm generated when you begin the program is depleted whenever you tell someone who does not understand how the mind works. You need that energy to get you started, so do not waste it on talking to other people, just do the action!

This program is based on scientific principles and you will receive in exact proportions the results you put into it. In other words, if you devote 50 percent of your time to the program, you will receive 50 percent results. If you devote 75 percent, you will receive 75 percent results. Whatever you put into something, you always receive back rewards proportional to your amount of effort.

CHAPTER 17

Beyond the Mind

We have explored the physical mechanics of aging and the mental mechanics of aging. Now we must explore beyond the mind, beyond the senses. We must go beyond what we can see, what we can hear, what we can taste, what we smell, and what we can feel.

Now that we have realized that age is but a state of mind, we also realize that we are much more than our bodies, much more than our emotions, and much more than our minds. There is a greater "something" that is eternal of which we are a part.

You were created in the image of God. God is life, and in that life that is God there are no years. Life has within itself the law of continuity. There is no "age" to deal with.

Your real life is the life you are living on a spiritual level. The body is not the governor of that life, but that life governs the body. Life really is an animating principle of the body. The body is not a law unto your life, your life is a law unto your body.

The mind is a window

You may think of your mind as a window looking into the greater consciousness that we call God, Creator. This window in your mind up to this time has been so dirty, so caked with negativity, false concepts, and erroneous attitudes that it has been impossible to see through it, to realize there is something greater than ourselves.

As you begin to cleanse this window by changing your negative emotions, attitudes, and concepts to positive vibrant thoughts, you begin to become aware of a greater "something." You realize that there is no way that you can have this perfect body and mind by accident. Something must have had an idea of the greatness within you. That perfection, that greatness is in the center of your being.

The center of your being is always in harmony, always at peace and in balance. It is much like the hub of a wheel. Although the wheels go around, the hub is always centered, always harmonious. So it is with the center of your being. As you practice the principles of life presented in this book, you will begin to contact the center of your being, that place within you that is always in perfect harmony, no matter what the worldly turmoil may be around you. Once you get centered within your being, it will not matter what is going on around you, you will be at perfect peace, without fear, anxiety, worries, or tension of any kind. This then, is indeed a "heaven on earth."

See the real you

Right now, at this moment, go to the nearest mirror. Take a good long hard look at yourself, not at the image in the mirror, but deep into your eyes, into your very soul. This is the real you, peering out of your eyes. This is the person your creative principle intended for you to be, not the image in the mirror.

You are not simply your body, you are not simply your mind, you are much greater than these. Get in touch with the inner being within you by becoming aware that it is there. That's all you have to do to contact it, become aware that it is there.

Perhaps you have thoughts such as, "If this had only been twenty years sooner, it's just too late for me now." Or you may be a person past the years of working and raising your family. You may be a widow or widower in a rest home. No matter what so-called age you are now, no matter what your circumstance, you can change it *now!* For you and you alone have control over your mind and you are the only one who can change it. Change yourself and you change your world.

Decide right now to be that creative being your Creator intended for you to be. Realize at this very moment you can and must take action that will change your world for you. You have one tremendous advantage that the other creatures do not have. You have your incredible mind. But even more than that, you have the most priceless gift of all: *the power of choice!*

The master secret of this universe and the key that

changes your world for you is *awareness* of this, the greatest of all gifts. If you are not aware of it, it is of no use to you. The only thing you have do to is to realize it, and that puts the principle into motion.

The simple techniques in this book show you that if you are persistent, you can not only turn off your age, but your world will also be the most totally new and tremendous world you could ever have imagined.

Youth is a state of mind

Begin now by the deep inner realization that youth is a state of mind. The youth we speak of in this book is not merely a physical thing of youthful good looks and supple knees; no, it is much more than that. It is a temper of your mind, a quality of your imagination, a vigor of your emotions. It is a freshness of the deep wellspring of life. Youth means predominance of courage over timidity, of the love of adventure over the comfort of security. This often exists in a mature man much more than in a boy of twenty or in a mature woman much more than in a girl of sixteen.

No one grows old by merely living a number of years. People grow old only by deserting their ideals, losing their curiosity for living. To give up enthusiasm wrinkles the soul. Worry, doubt, self-distrust, fear, desperation—these are the age-makers that turn your spirit back to the dust.

Yes, indeed, youth is a state of mind rather than a sum of years. At this very moment you can begin the positive actions that will turn off your age. *Begin now!*

"His flesh shall be fresher than a child's: he shall return to the days of his youth." (Job 33:25)

Also Available: Think Slim–Be Slim

Another popular book by Elsye Birkinshaw outlines a proven 21-day plan for perfect weight control and a lifelong ideal body image. At bookstores or health food stores or from the publisher: Woodbridge Press, Box 6189, Santa Barbara, CA 93111. Send $5 US funds, including postage and handling.

Cassette tapes available

The following are examples of cassette tapes available (see address below) to help you recondition your mind so you can more easily turn off your age, and to teach you how to relax. It has been found in our classes that learning time has been cut in half by the use of the tapes.

Tape No. 3

Side 1: *Sound of the Bells* (learning how to relax with background of five bells, the bells affecting the subconscious in totally unexpected ways—based on a oriental theory of musical harmonics that makes relaxation a total experience)

Side 2: *Sound of the Bells* (helping you to visualize your ideal body image)

Tape No. 6

Side 1: *Goals* (using your creative imagination to picture any goal you wish to achieve)

Side 2: *Quiet Pool* (a deep relaxation to help you reach the depths of your inner knowledge and develop self-confidence)

Tape No. 8

Side 1: *A Forest Clearing* (to help you to develop your creative imagination and expand your awareness of yourself)

Side 2: *Who Are You?* (know thyself; that is the secret of the ages)

Tape No. 10

Side 1: *Turn Off Your Age* (you were not meant to grow old, you only allow it to happen because you don't know how to stop it)
Side 2: *Progressive Relaxation* (sound of bells in background) (A fundamental technique to create a brain-cell impression to detect the difference between tension and relaxation)

Tape 11

Side 1: *Principle of Forgiveness* (This mental exercise will cleanse your mind of negative debris)
Side 2: *Break the Chains that Bind You* (Do not live out your whole life by being a prisoner in your own mind, in a prison of negative beliefs, erroneous concepts. Break the chain of false attitudes)

Tape 12

Side 1: *In Search of* (this tape attempts to answer the soul-searching question, "Who Am I?")
Side 2: *This Is Reality* (What is reality? Is it the things we see, hear, touch, smell or taste? Or is there something beyond the senses?)

The above tapes are exclusively for helping you to learn the technique of relaxation and expand your creative imagination so you may have help in "turning off your age."

They are not produced or distributed by the publishers of this book and are listed here only as a convenience for the reader.

They may be ordered directly from: Seminars of Self-Awareness, Box 202, Pinedale, California 93650, at $12 for each tape plus $1.00 for postage and handling in the U.S. For foreign orders, please send international money order plus the applicable airmail postage to your country, in U.S. dollars. The tapes weigh 1½ oz. each.

For a listing of these and other subjects, send a card with your address to the address just above.